Hard to Kill

Master the Mindset to Maximize Your Years

Jaime Seeman, M.D.

Published by
Fit & Fabulous, LLC

For Kimberlee Loutzenhiser, you taught me more in death than in life and your ripples will last forever.

Table of Contents

Introduction

From the minute we're born, the only guarantee in life is death. This may sound like a harsh reality, but as an OBGYN, it's one of the things I think about every time I deliver a baby. I also think about the possibilities—who they will become, what they will achieve, and the impact they will have on the world. Each one of us leaves a legacy when we're no longer here—a legacy that tells our own story about the lives we touched during our time on earth. Greatness is the ability to inspire the people around you. I want to inspire you so that you can leave a legacy that inspires others.

The guarantee of death is what makes our time on earth so precious. It's a lesson I learned after a traumatic life event that became the catalyst to change for myself and my family. It's why everyone needs to create a quality life and why I want to give you the skills to create that life with whatever time you're given. After all, time and energy are our most valuable assets, and the best way to maximize them is by becoming someone who is hard to kill.

There are five pillars of health needed to achieve a quality life and become hard to kill: nutrition, movement, sleep, stress resilience, and environment. You can't neglect one pillar for another; they must all work together. I'll provide detailed explanations about each pillar of health so that you'll gain an in-depth knowledge of each one and learn how to incorporate them into your own life. I'll also provide a Hard to Kill 30-day Challenge so that you can start right away.

Being hard to kill is more than just staving off illness or disease. It's waking up each day with a burning desire to want the life you have and everything it encompasses—your body, your family, and all the circumstances that come with it. Within that structure, you learn how to be successful in all areas of your life: physical, intellectual, financial, spiritual, and social. Being hard to kill is a slow journey that takes time. It's a continuum in which you can move forward and backward on any given day. Like most transformations, not everyone in your current circle of influence will be accepting or ready to follow you. It doesn't mean you have to revert back to previous ways or make an immediate change forward, but you may have to eventually let go of some people who aren't willing to support you.

Being hard to kill isn't for everybody; it's a lifestyle often lived in the margins. But the margins of life are where some of the biggest influencers and thought leaders historically reside. Once you start your journey, you'll find an endless network of people, like me, who are willing and eager to meet you at any point and in any capacity along the way. Even though I'm a physician, my white coat hasn't provided me with a fast pass to becoming hard to kill. I've had to work on it over many years, and I hope my experiences will serve as an example of how to implement the Hard to Kill principles.

Becoming hard to kill isn't a quick fix that happens overnight. It's a life-long mentality, and the fastest way to get there is slowly. I'll teach you the skills necessary to take ownership of the things you can control and how to truly let go of the things you can't. This will give you the ability to have a mindset in which you can select your thoughts just like you select the clothes you wear each day. This ability is the equivalent of a superpower, but a superpower that you must cultivate and practice over time. Ultimately, if you want control of your life, you must learn how to control your mind.

So, if you feel bored, stuck, stale, have become uninterested and uninspired, or have success in some areas of your life but have neglected other areas, then you are ready to become hard to kill. Nobody else is going to save you; it's something you have to do for yourself. But it's attainable for anyone willing to work for it. My real hope is that once you've obtained the hard to kill mindset, you'll share it and help teach it to others, because a ripple effect is how we truly change the world. I want to help you create something that lasts. I want to help you create your legacy. I want to move through this together, so that you can make the most of this precious life you've been given. I want you to use your time and energy on earth to become someone who is hard to kill because your inspired, new way of living will help turn the tides of change in the world. Set aside the emotion, drama, and attitude. The solution to healing starts within you.

Chapter 1
No One is Coming to Save You

Youth is Lost on the Young

One of the important principles to understand and adopt about the hard to kill mentality is the notion that no one is coming to save you—the only person who can save you is yourself. It took me a lot of years, unnecessary health issues, and a traumatic life event to embrace this fact as part of my hard to kill journey.

I grew up in the Midwest as a three-sport athlete, straight-A student, and a natural leader. Keeping busy and staying active was how I excelled. My mom was a nurse and the leader of our family, so a career in healthcare was my goal from a young age. Every activity I pursued came easily, whether it was school or sports—I never had to work extra hard to find success.

The first big challenge in my life happened as a Division I

collegiate athlete, as a pitcher for the University of Nebraska —Lincoln (UNL). Not only was it suddenly difficult to balance the demands of school and still excel on the field, but my Exercise Science program was eliminated from the university. In a panic, I switched to biology, only to switch again a few months later to journalism, with the thought of being a news anchor. Before I started journalism classes, the university created a Nutrition, Exercise, and Health Science program. My mom had encouraged me to become a physician —something she wished she had done—because she recognized my desire to help people. So as an aspiring physician, the new program was the perfect path for me to pursue.

Despite the fact I was studying nutrition and exercise, I battled an internal struggle as a female athlete. I gave no thought to food—we were always told what to eat and when to eat it—and weight lifting was a critical component to my sport. I embraced that physical challenge and was a two-time Lifter of the Year at UNL. However, I started to realize how society viewed the female athletic body. I was always physically large with big legs, living in a decade where "thin" and "skinny" were all I saw on magazine covers and TV. Weight lifting equated to masculinity, and you couldn't be masculine and feminine or sexy at the same time. I felt a divide to be one or the other, rather than smart, pretty, and physically strong all at the same time. People often commented on the size of my leg muscles. It never felt like a compliment, and I prayed for the day I could stop playing sports and my legs would magically melt away forever. I also started dating in college. By God's grace, I met my husband, Ben, who was playing college football at the time, and there was a stigma that a female shouldn't be able to lift more weight than a male. As I entered this vulnerable period in my life, I always minimized my physical strength in hopes it would not intimidate a potential suitor, including Ben.

Even my female teammates influenced my body image views. Softball was a sport in which dirt covered your face rather than makeup. But I still wanted to look feminine, especially when our games were televised. So, I'd curl my hair and put on makeup. I wanted to look good while playing, but my teammates chastised me. I questioned whether I could really be all the different parts at once. By the time I graduated, I vowed to never lift weights again. I wanted to fit the "mold" of what a smart, feminine woman should look like —and it didn't include large leg muscles or being able to lift heavy weights. I felt like I had to be a smaller, quieter version of myself, especially when around others.

I had a break following graduation in 2007 when I was waitlisted for medical school. It enabled me to plan my wedding (I even worked in a bridal shop). Shortly after being married, I was accepted into medical school at the University of Nebraska Medical Center. Once again, I struggled with the transition. Instead of the constant physical activity as a collegiate athlete, I sat in a classroom five days a week with tests every Saturday. Despite having a degree in nutrition and exercise, I didn't know how to eat right, I counted calories just to maintain a "normal" body weight, and I had anxiety from the pressure to be competitive in medical school. My body composition changed, and I had new concerns with my body image. My strong body was becoming softer by the day as I ditched the weights in favor of cardio and trying to count calories.

The Struggle is Real

During medical school, Ben and I decided to start a family. We struggled to get pregnant. After years of birth control, my menstrual cycles were irregular and I was diagnosed with Polycystic Ovary Syndrome (PCOS), which is a hormonal disorder. With the help of medication, I finally became pregnant but failed my pregnancy glucose test. Thankfully, we were blessed with our first daughter, Breklyn, in August of 2011. However, I was soon diagnosed with postpartum hypothyroidism and required medication. But that wasn't enough to change my poor eating and nutrition habits. I was a new mom, a medical student, the wife of a police officer on night shifts, and I was just trying to survive.

In medical school I fell in love with Obstetrics and Gynecology. It was the perfect blend of performing surgeries and delivering life into the world, as well as helping women through every decade of life. After completing medical school, I matched to an OBGYN residency program. Little did I know at the time I made that choice I would have three daughters of my own that would drive my purpose in life even further.

Ben and I got pregnant again, and our second daughter, Sienna, was born in July 2013. Suddenly, I realized how much weight I'd gained with my first two pregnancies, and I desperately wanted my pre-pregnancy body back. I thought I needed to eat less and move more, so I bought a treadmill, set it up in our living room, and immediately signed up for a half-marathon. I had never been a runner, in fact, I despised it. But I knew my competitive nature would be a driving force. I trained on my treadmill for months and completed my first half-marathon in under two hours—1 hour and 57 minutes. Even though I had accomplished my goal, I didn't see the changes in body composition I had hoped for. Instead, I was chronically fatigued, working 80 hours a week as a medical resident to pay off my student debt from medical school, and had a newborn and a two-year-old. I was a working mother trying to care for my family at the cost of neglecting my own health. My husband was working nights and weekends as a police officer, supporting us the best he could.

The following year, my best friend Kimberlee convinced me to get pregnant at the same time with both of our third children. She had two daughters as well, so our girls were ages one, two, three, and four. We found out we were pregnant three weeks apart and joked that one of us was bound to have a boy who would be terrorized by all the girls. As excited as I was to go through pregnancy with my best friend, deep down I still struggled with eating, not exercising the right way, and with being a mom and living a busy life. We were just trying to survive, or so I thought.

A Life with Purpose and Passion

In January 2015, Kimberlee came down with a respiratory infection. She went to her doctor, who treated it, but it didn't go away. Over the next 6-8 weeks it got worse, and she steadily grew sicker. In March 2015, she was suddenly hospitalized in the ICU as doctors tried to determine her illness. I visited her every day and watched her health decline—first as they sedated her and inserted a breathing tube, and then as she lost her baby boy, Jack. I agonized over how we'd tell her when she eventually woke up. Doctors finally diagnosed Kimberlee with a rare fungal infection that was ravishing her body, but by then it was too late. Days later, she succumbed to the infection and passed away.

I questioned everything in that moment—the doctors' inability to save a healthy 29-year-old, my own ability as an OBGYN to help women, not to mention my ability as a mother. But it's during our worst tragedies that we gain the most, and what Kimberlee taught me on that day is our time on earth is never guaranteed. I made a vow to her and to myself that I would live my life with a different purpose and passion.

In June 2015, our third daughter was born—Kimber Lee. Three weeks later Kimberlee would have been due with Jack, which was devastating, especially for her husband and two daughters. When you lose a loved one, every milestone is hard to endure. During those days and weeks, life seemed so uncertain, unfair, and uncontrollable. I knew the risk for developing postpartum depression because I'd had it following my first two pregnancies. I felt the need to take action and have a sense of physical control to prevent depression from setting in. So, seven days after giving birth, I signed up at a boxing gym. Breast milk leaked through my sports bra, I could hardly hold my bladder, and my body was the worst version of myself I'd ever seen. But I had made a vow that I was determined to keep, and that day became the starting point for what I knew I could become—hard to kill.

Fit & Fabulous

A year later, I graduated residency and started my career as a private practice OBGYN. I had some labs checked and discovered not only did I still have hypothyroidism, but I had developed pre-diabetes too. I was shocked and embarrassed that I had gotten to a point where I was living with preventable medical conditions. It was time for me to start walking the walk as a health care provider. Needing to again take action, I dove into literature to learn how to reverse these conditions. Ben had also been struggling with migraines, so we decided to make changes together, starting with our diet. We began with Whole30, then paleo, and by the spring of 2016 we had adopted the ketogenic (keto) diet. For the first time since college, the weight effortlessly came off, my energy returned, the nighttime fatigue disappeared, and my brain worked more efficiently. Ben's symptoms vanished too.

At that time, the keto diet was not widely accepted by the public or the health community, and I lived in an isolated space both as a person and as a physician. Even as I dove into research and data, the only information I found was that it helped epileptic children. Regardless, Ben and I continued our keto lifestyle, even sharing it with family and friends. I slowly started connecting with other providers in the low carb space and shared the information with my patients. The results were amazing and mirrored the findings from pioneers researching ketogenic therapy and its impact on preventable medical conditions.

The top three causes of death are cardiovascular disease—including diabetes—cancer, and neurologic disorders. I wanted to prevent my patients, family, friends, and myself from developing one of these conditions. I wanted to make a large impact on my community and even the world, but I'd need to speak out about it to do so. I decided to complete a two-year fellowship in integrative medicine to fully understand and immerse myself in traditional and complementary forms of medicine. I'd also need to become accountable to the world and share my journey so that anyone—a struggling mom, diabetic, or another physician—had a place to connect. One night while sitting on my couch I created a social media profile. Although it was a declaration without evidence, I wanted a name that best described whom I wanted to become: Dr. Fit & Fabulous. I made a commitment to live up to that name.

Game Changer

I made amazing progress with my weight loss and symptoms, but I still felt physically weak and soft. In March 2018, I started weight lifting again, and all of my former body image concerns came rushing back. I didn't want to lift but knew it was the only way to make the changes I wanted. I also combined it with a more carnivore-based keto lifestyle. I committed to both the diet and lifting, waking up every morning at 4:30 am to go to the gym. I knew if I didn't pay myself first, then I couldn't take care of anybody else. Day by day, my body morphed into its best composition I'd ever experienced. I also had physical power like I'd never had in my adult life. My pre-diabetes was gone, my hypothyroidism was gone, and I operated at a whole new level.

That same year, a scrub tech in the operating room at the hospital mentioned to me in passing that I should try out for a TV show called *Titan Games*. I hadn't heard of it, and when I looked it up online, it reminded me of the show *American Gladiator*, which I grew up watching. As a little girl, I wanted to be just like the female gladiator, Diamond. But that image didn't fit a thirty-something physician and mom. Not to mention the physical requirements listed on the application— I was too far removed from being a collegiate athlete to ever accomplish that level of strength. The self-doubt was all-consuming.

For months, thoughts of *Titan Games* gnawed at me. I had declared who I was—Dr. Fit & Fabulous—and I didn't want external forces to perpetuate the paradigm that a doctor and mother of three couldn't also be strong enough to compete. But I knew myself well enough to know that if I couldn't compete at the level I wanted, then I didn't want to compete at all. Finally, in the fall of 2019, I submitted my application. After all, what was the worst that could happen?

Titan Games showcases everyday heroes, so the application included a video about my personal story and clips of me at my job as well as performing physical strength tests. It was the first time I experienced the fusion of me as a doctor and as an "American Gladiator." I started watching all the episodes of season one of *Titan Games* to see what they had to do. I ramped up my workouts and trained on my own. Nobody except my husband knew I had applied, not even my mother. But days, weeks, and months went by, and I never heard from the show, so I assumed I hadn't been good enough.

Right before Christmas 2019, I received a phone call that I was being considered for the show and should clear my schedule for three weeks in February just in case. But first, I had to compete in a combine. In January 2020, I flew to California where I competed against 100 other people for a spot on the show. I was immediately humbled by the contestants and their inspiring stories of defeat, death, and tragedy. There were many contestants much younger and more physically powerful than me. I was flooded with insecurities and questioned why I had been chosen to compete.

Even though it had been more than 12 years since I had participated in a strength competition, I gave it my best and exceeded my expectations. It was invigorating! A flame was lit that day. I had a realization that even though you go through phases in life, you don't have to give away any part of yourself. I was ready to compete and prayed my performance would earn me that chance. I left the combine knowing only that 16 men and women would be chosen. I had to wait again. The next week I received a phone call—I had been given a spot on the show! I had one week to prepare before flying out to Atlanta for filming. I was able to tell my family and friends I was going to be on a TV show, but not the name of it. Guesses included *Naked and Afraid, American Ninja Warrior*, and even a medical show.

I arrived in Atlanta and quickly realized I was an underdog. Most of the contestants were younger and some were currently competing athletes, including Olympians. But it gave me a chance to prove that age is just a number and you shouldn't back down from a challenge just because the odds don't seem in your favor. The opportunity that came with wearing the *Titan Games* uniform was priceless. I could show my three girls it was okay to do something that terrifies you, and that you can be smart, physically strong, and feel beautiful all at the same time. I wasn't just representing me; I was representing moms and people who feel like they've lost their former selves. That uniform embraced the idea that you could be all things at once. The only person stopping you from anything you want in life is you.

The *Titan Games* arena was a small studio full of lights, cameras, smoke, and obstacles made up of items you've never seen before. With my family in the studio and the whole world watching on TV, I was overwhelmed with the fear that I was going to lose and quickly be done. I didn't want to disappoint anyone, including myself. I stayed focused and won my first two competitions. I moved on to regionals, but lost, which was very heavy emotionally. I'd have to fight my way back into the winner's bracket, so I focused on what I could control, which was my mindset.

During regionals, my favorite moment was the barrel toss competition. I was tethered to my opponent, and we each had to toss five 50-pound barrels over a barrier while pulling against each other. It's one thing to face your opponent, but I couldn't see her or the scoreboard, so I had no idea who was winning. Instead, I had tunnel-vision and a strategy I knew I needed to execute. When I tossed the fifth barrel, the studio erupted in cheers and pyrotechnics exploded around the arena. Then I saw my face on the large screen and Dwayne "The Rock" Johnson, who hosted the show, congratulated and hugged me. I was completely out of breath but ran to my family. They were so excited, and my girls even flexed their biceps in a show of solidarity.

I finished in the top six of all women on the show. That may seem insignificant compared to what I do every day as a physician, but it felt amazing to step into something completely new, have a plan, and then execute on that plan. It fulfilled a dream just to be selected for the show, but I competed my best and showed the world that a mom and physician could also be a Titan.

Strong Beauty Queen

During the months I waited to hear back from *Titan Games*, a new opportunity arose. My neighbor, a former Miss South Dakota, suggested I run for Mrs. Nebraska. I didn't even know there was a pageant system for married women! Once again, my first thought was that a doctor and mother of three couldn't possibly wear a swimsuit and walk on stage in front of thousands of people. My body certainly didn't fit the mold of a beauty queen, and I had no experience in the pageant industry. But just like with *Titan Games*, the thought of competing in a beauty pageant simmered in the back of my mind. It would be a great way to break the mold that a beauty pageant was simply about a pretty face or a certain body type. I also learned that the interview portion accounts for 50%, so it would be a good platform to spread my message about preventative health. In December 2019—the same month I found out about *Titan Games*—I submitted an application to compete for Mrs. Nebraska.

The pageant was scheduled for April 2020, but I was forced to focus on *Titan Games* first. It wasn't until I had come back from filming the show that I was able to finally realize I had to compete in a beauty pageant just two months later. So, I hit the ground running. I hired a pageant coach and practiced walking in 5 3/4-inch heels—quite the opposite of *Titan Games*. I was confident in the interview portion, but I wasn't used to wearing fancy dresses, parading in swimsuits, or walking in really, really high heels. During all my prep, I constantly reminded and reassured myself it was okay that I didn't look like a typical pageant contestant. I had big muscles and multiple academic degrees, and my mission was to ignore the stigma and redefine the title.

In March 2020, the pandemic hit, and the pageant was rescheduled for August. With the world in lockdown, it would have been easy to use it as an excuse to shut down, quit, and feel "small" again. Instead, I used it to reinforce my purpose and not let it stop me from continuing to grow and excel. I stayed focused on what was in front of me. The pageant was finally held in August, and the competition was really impressive. The women were all incredibly talented, beautiful, and articulate. My biggest obstacle was my insecurity of not looking like the other contestants as I walked across the stage and not representing the paradigm of a beauty queen. Instead, I represented the duality of eloquence and strength while spreading my message of health. I wondered how many lives I could change with that message by wearing the crown. During the evening gown competition, we drew interview questions that had been submitted by other contestants. My question was, "What is the best thing that's ever happened in your life?" The answer was meeting my husband. He's been so supportive every step of the way, and I wouldn't have my family, career, or accomplishments without him.

I made it into the top five of the pageant, and at that stage of the competition the point system went back to zero and the on-stage interview determined the final outcome. All five women were on stage and could hear each other's questions and answers. My final question was, "If crowned, what impact would you want to have?" My answer was that I wanted to inspire all Nebraskans to take control of their health because it's not something that can be bought. Every individual has to do it for themselves. After the interview, I felt I had delivered the best answer I could and waited for the judges' decision. When they finally announced the winner and I heard my name, it literally took my breath away. To win something when you feel like you're against all the odds was an incredible success. Having my girls in the audience to see it was one of my proudest moments as a mom. It was also validating that the world was open to the idea of what I represented—someone well-spoken, physically strong, academically smart, and full of grit and tenacity. But winning Mrs. Nebraska wasn't just my accomplishment. It represented much more than myself. It was a win for everyone who's helped along the way, for my friends, my husband, and my strong girls. We all won that night.

The pageant was such a surreal experience. The middle of a pandemic seemed like the perfect time to spread my message of resilience through nutrition and movement. Although the pandemic prevented me from in-person appearances, I was still able to appear on video conference and speak to schools, give radio interviews, and I even wore my sash and crown while participating in the 50 Mile March to support veteran non-profit organizations.

I went on to compete in the Mrs. America pageant in Las Vegas, which had been rescheduled for March 2021. I finished in the top 15 and was really proud of myself. As a competitive person, I always have an expectation to give my best effort, but you also can't win everything. If you avoid failure, you will avoid success. Unfortunately, my message seemed to fall on deaf ears as I realized the pageant industry as a whole still wasn't ready for physically strong, powerful women. Like most industries, politics seemed to prevail.

Despite that, the experience fueled my fire. I didn't need the Mrs. America crown and sash to make a big impact. I had set out on a divine path and nothing was going to get in my way. It was like a giant ball had been set in motion. The *Titan Games* and the pageants happened in succession by fate—I wasn't bored, looking for something to pass the time. Those two events showed me that I was capable of being both a Titan and a beauty queen. I was finally living as my authentic self.

Save Yourself

The number one thing I learned from Kimberlee's death, the *Titan Games*, and the beauty pageants, is that nobody was coming to save me. Nobody could do the work for me. Nobody could fix my feelings of being stuck despite knowing there was something bigger and better within me. With the competitions, I went after two things that seemed impossible for a physician and a mother in her late thirties. Both of those events were monumental in showing me that my only limit was me. You don't have to win something to gain power and perspective, you just have to go after it. Once I accepted that I had to save myself, then I was able to move forward. When you stop making excuses, put your own insecurities aside, and ignore what society says you should be, then you can become powerful beyond measure. This is a scary thought for most people, but in life we regularly restrict our potential through self-limiting thoughts and behaviors.

We all have to be accountable for where we are currently and where we are going, especially when it comes to our health. You'll never feel completely ready, and there is never a perfect time to start. You are ready right now. The time to start is right now. Confidence is only built through action, and your internal dialogue is what drives that action. Telling yourself that you're ready, now, is the first step to becoming hard to kill.

Chapter 2
The 5 Pillars of Health

Definition of Health
When you think of the word "health," what does it take to achieve it? Being physically active? Not eating junk food? Sleeping eight hours a night? According to the *Merriam-Webster Dictionary*, the definition of health is, "the condition of being well or free from disease," or "the overall condition of someone's body or mind." While these are both true, having health means you are able to do what you want physically, mentally, and spiritually with whom you choose in whatever time you're given. Your health manifests in your physical appearance and also in your performance. In other words, having health means you're hard to kill in this moment.

A lot of things can be bought in this world, but your health isn't one of them. Nobody can improve your health for you or do the work to achieve it. I took my health for granted for many years. Through my struggles, I realized there were five areas in my life that had to be addressed to optimize how I feel and function. I'm going to introduce you to these 5 pillars of health that I believe everyone needs to address. Once practiced and mastered, you'll have the necessary tools to become hard to kill.

The most important form of health is physical. You only get one body and one brain. Imagine you're an expensive car. Everything you do to the car affects how it performs: how fast you drive, the type of fuel you use, and whether or not you have it serviced for maintenance. If you encounter problems, you can replace parts. You can even paint it a different color. But if you total the car, it's beyond repair. Unlike a car, you can't go to the dealer and just buy a new year and model for your body. Let's face it—many people take better care of their car than they do themselves. They have car wash memberships, digital reminders to change the oil, and even self-driving cars. But nothing—not even your car—is more valuable than you. There are almost 8 billion people in the world and your make and model is unique to *you*.

The field of medicine is amazing. I can perform surgery using anesthesia. My colleagues can transplant organs. We even know how to cure some cancers. But the field of medicine is also broken. Doctors are tired of it too. We are expected to see more patients, in less time, churning people through the hamster wheel. Most of your healthcare dollars are spent treating chronic conditions that may add some years to your life, but are they quality years? How many of those years are spent in and out of doctor's offices, hospitals, and pharmacies? You can't stop or reverse the aging process, (although smart people are working on that), but you can maximize the quality of your years regardless.

When it comes to managing chronic disease, money and politics are always at play. Although doctors have their patients' health at heart, political systems and "big pharma" don't. The only foreseeable solution to the healthcare crisis is self-accountability. You need to take ownership of everything you can control. I will help you realize you're powerful beyond measure, but you'll have to physically and mentally share that power with the rest of the world—you can't be powerful alone.

In 2020, a global pandemic swept the world. Its devastation revealed the importance of metabolic health. Society learned that people who have metabolic disease such as type 2 diabetes, high blood pressure, high visceral fat, and other preventable chronic conditions are at much higher risk of severe disease and even death. Despite this revelation, the message was widely ignored, especially by the country's leaders, most of whom don't lead healthy lifestyles themselves. During a crisis, people survive because they do simple tasks to stay alive—things they can control. Yet there was a huge absence of information about the simple things people could have controlled during the pandemic to improve health. The pandemic messaging was more problem-driven than solution-driven. The message needs to be clear: your body is an intricate machine at a cellular level and will take care of you if you take care of it in return.

Simply "looking" healthy is only a veil. I looked healthy but had pre-diabetes and hypothyroidism, so you have to be cautious about judging health based on external appearances only. Remember, performance and other key biometrics should be used for proper health optimization. Following my fellowship in integrative medicine, I held group coaching to help people with diet and nutrition. Through this work, I quickly learned that you could eat the most optimal diet, but if you weren't moving correctly, sleeping well, developing your mindset, and reducing stress, you'd never achieve a true state of health. That's why all five pillars of health are so important. It's okay to just start with one, but eventually you'll need to ensure all five are strong in order to become hard to kill.

Pillar 1: Nutrition

Everywhere you turn, you're bombarded with diet culture. People have walk-in pantries, multiple refrigerators, and food delivered with one tap of a phone app. The concept of a family meal is rare because everyone lives a fast-paced life in order not to fall behind. Lifestyle dictates eating habits, and people easily succumb to foods of convenience without thinking about the effect on their bodies. Yet the one thing that can have the biggest impact on health in the shortest amount of time is what you eat.

Humans live very differently from our ancestors. Early humans were hunter-gatherers who had to kill wild animals for protein and fat. If they didn't get a kill, then they had to fast or forage for fruits and vegetables. They literally cultivated their diet. Today, it's rare for someone to eat in a way that mimics our ancestors. Every home in America has pantries full of boxed, bagged, and jarred food with a long list of ingredients on the label. Unfortunately, it's no different at most medical offices and hospitals, including my own. We need to stop accepting this as normal and reframe the narrative. Instead of food as entertainment, we need to think of food as fuel. I'll teach you some simple rules to take control of your diet so you feel satisfied but not deprived.

Food addiction is a problem in society, especially binging. People condemn drug, alcohol, and sex addiction but don't think twice about eating a dozen donuts or supersized fast-food meal. As a child, I hid food in my room and couldn't wait to be alone to eat it. Even now, being alone with food is problematic for me. My pregnancies were excuses to eat whatever I wanted. I also spent years counting calories—even counting individual goldfish crackers—or snacking on a box of Hot Tamales candy because it had a heart healthy label. But this stigma and view of food can change. No food is inherently bad—it's usually the dose that makes the poison.

The first pillar will also explore the politics of food and nutrition policies. Every day, consumers vote with their dollars and where they spend them. Food manufacturers know their highly-processed foods are addictive, cheap, and readily available. On the flip side, social media floods our news feeds with diet options: vegan, carnivore, Mediterranean, cleanses, and fasting. You're not alone in feeling overwhelmed and confused. I have a nutrition degree and used to count goldfish crackers!

Your body is designed to consume whole foods with the nutrients necessary to fuel every one of its systems. If an animal at the zoo isn't fed a diet found in its natural habitat, it will die. Nature always gets it right and gives us instructions for our genes to follow—an internal blueprint. People shouldn't try to outsmart nature. Just because we have the knowledge, resources, and technology to do so, neglecting what nature has provided will lead to disaster. There's a complex symbiotic relationship at play in your body, and food either feeds or fights disease. Nutrition is an ever-evolving world, but it's a relatively simple pillar to accomplish as long as you remember one simple principle: food is medicine. If you eat better, you can avoid many chronic diseases.

Pillar 2: Movement

All movement is good, but not all movement is created equal. Movement to gain muscle is the most important kind. I had a hard time accepting this as a female athlete because of the fear of looking less feminine. But muscle is a critical organ of longevity, especially for women. It helps you become hard to kill for a long time.

Muscle is a use it or lose it organ that has been overlooked by both the medical and fitness industries for far too long. Over-promoting cardio has come at a cost. Although cardio is healthy, spending an hour on the treadmill or elliptical machine isn't as beneficial as a session of resistance training on a consistent basis. Once you gain muscle, you must continue to develop it so you don't lose it. I'll teach you some strategies for gaining muscle, which is such a critical component to the aging process. Most people aren't "over fat" they are "under muscled".

Pillar 3: Sleep

Do you know how to sleep? It's more than just lying down and closing your eyes. And for those who think, "I'll sleep when I'm dead," then you'll be easy to kill. Unfortunately, most people abuse sleep and don't prioritize waking rest. Our culture praises work and overachievement so much that stopping to rest is perceived as lazy. Rest doesn't have to mean taking a nap. Rest can be as simple as calming your mind during waking hours, which is necessary to complete difficult tasks. Think of rest like a light switch.

Knowing when to turn it off, turn it on, or dim it can make a world of difference for your health.

Your body is a receiver of light. The absence or presence of light is what sets your circadian rhythm—your connection to nature. Sleep is the only time your body repairs, regenerates, and makes the hormones necessary for its systems to function properly. In fact, what you often perceive as daytime problems and stressors are actually the result of nighttime problems due to poor sleep hygiene. Similar to needing the right environment to work, you need the right environment for optimal sleep. Noisy, warm bedrooms full of technology interfere with the body's circadian rhythm. Smart phones are the biggest culprits, radiating even small amounts of light that your eyes can sense. I'll share some simple steps to improve your sleep hygiene and help make you harder to kill.

Pillar 4: A Resilient Mindset

Stress seems to be at an all-time high and unavoidable at every turn. But most people have an inaccurate view toward stress. When you're stressed, it simply means you care about the situation. If you can welcome stress and use it toward your advantage, then you'll have a skill that most people never learn.

This pillar will teach you resilience in mind, body, and spirit. It will focus on controlling your mind so that your body isn't physically impacted in a negative way. When you learn how to respond to daily stressors, you become mentally and physically unbreakable. It's not an easy skill to master and takes lots of practice, but you'll be able to select your thoughts and let the negative ones go.

I will discuss the following mindfulness techniques: meditation, breathwork, and self-talk, which is important because the language you use sets the tone every day. I will also discuss physical resilience and a multifaceted approach that includes modalities such as yoga, stretching, and cold and heat therapy. All of these methods nurture the parasympathetic nervous system, also known as the "rest and digest" system, critical for stress recovery. Finally, I'll discuss spiritual resilience and how you can connect with your own higher calling. It's important to always think about your purpose in life, connecting with people, and the ripples you can make in the world as a result of living a life of passion.

Pillar 5: Environment

This pillar encompasses all of the people, places, and things you interact with every day: your city, your home, people, and even the products you use and consume. Every aspect of your environment impacts your mental, physical, and spiritual well-being. It's true that you become the five people you interact with the most, so it's important to audit that immediate circle on a regular basis. There could be people very close to you who are inadvertently sabotaging your efforts to become hard to kill. I'll teach you how to avoid this trap and connect with the hard to kill community so you have a circle of people who support you and can help you flourish.

The place where you live and work has an impact on your health. The materials used to build, paint, and decorate your home and office could be contributing factors. Even the fabric of your couch, blankets, or sheets might lead to problems. Items used in daily routines play a bigger role than people realize, especially plastics, fragrances, food chemicals, and pesticides. They all seem unavoidable, but you can reduce your exposure and create an environment for health so that you don't just survive, you thrive.

As you dive into the next five chapters, you'll have to decide which pillar makes the most sense for you to start your journey. Keep in mind, you won't accomplish them all at once. Even now, I don't follow all five pillars perfectly. It takes continuous work day in and day out. It may take you days, weeks, or years of small steps, but you will get there. Being hard to kill isn't a destination. It's a mindset and a way of living that you and I can do together. Regardless of how much time you have left, you'll spend it doing everything you've learned to be hard to kill.

Chapter 3
Pillar 1: Nutrition

Evolution of Food
Nutrition isn't the only aspect of health—there are four other pillars in the Hard to Kill plan. Nutrition is important because every time you put food into your mouth, you're either feeding or fighting disease. There's a sad reality that some people panic more over a cell phone about to die than they do about preventing their own early death. Multiple studies have shown that up to 84% of people couldn't function a day without their cell phone. Imagine if that many people cared about their diet. Wouldn't it be great if you could just hook yourself to a portable power bank? Unfortunately, there is no way around proper nutrition—no cheat codes and no hacks. The online world is an overwhelming database of information about what, how, and

when to eat. Instead of trying to decipher it all, you simply need to look at your genetic makeup.

Early humans had to hunt for food—a literal feast or famine. As their brains evolved and grew, their diet encompassed fatty fish, pastured animals, and a sprinkle of carbohydrates from plants, which looked nothing like their modern counterparts. Humans developed specific intestinal bacteria to accommodate these foods, which created the perfect symbiotic relationship that resulted in optimal health. Their reliance on animal-based food developed unique metabolic pathways that today help you digest protein and fat. Modern society shouldn't have manipulated nature and needs to find a way to return to this type of diet to improve health.

Go back to 13,000 years ago when humans domesticated animals and began growing grains, which reduced their reliance on hunting, fishing, and gathering. This trend started a revolution that would dramatically reduce health over time. When archeologists studied mummified Egyptian bodies, they found evidence of obesity, decayed teeth, and heart disease. Why? Because they ate mostly bread, cereals, fruits and vegetables, and only small amounts of fish and poultry— similar to the "plant-based diets" that are popular today.

As agriculture progressed, populations increased, leading to more dense living conditions. Contaminated food, water, and soil led to widespread disease. Although modern sanitation and clean water have greatly helped, advancement and technology come at a cost. People can now abundantly store food and never have to leave home to get it. We expend very little energy with our modern lifestyles—vastly different than the energy expended by our ancestors to chase down a buffalo, kill it, prepare it, eat it, and make it last for an entire winter.

The Politics of Food

Then in the 1950s, society took another major turn. President Dwight D. Eisenhower had a heart attack on Friday, September 23rd, 1955, while playing golf in Denver, Colorado. He first attributed his discomfort to a hamburger he'd eaten for lunch. Panic ensued as the country searched for answers as to what caused his heart attack. Heart disease plagued the world and served as the leading cause of death among men. A witch hunt ensued, led and paid for by political and special interest groups. Scientists wanted to blame fat and hang it at the stake. The leading theory called the "diet-heart hypothesis" was established by an American physiologist named Ancel Keys who said dietary fat, cholesterol, and coronary artery disease were causally related —fat and cholesterol cause coronary artery disease. He failed to acknowledge that correlation doesn't automatically mean causation. An analogy is sharks and ice cream. During summer months, there is a rise in ice cream sales. There is also a rise in shark attacks. Does this mean ice cream sales cause shark attacks? No, it simply means there are more people swimming in the ocean during summer months who also buy ice cream.

Keys didn't account for several other factors, such as cigarette smoking, which was on the rise, and diets high in sugar, which were more prevalent. In fact, most diets high in fat are also high in sugar. That combo is like a drug that always keeps you coming back for more. (Personally, I've never met a donut I didn't like.) In the 1960s, the Sugar Research Foundation funded studies at Harvard University to refute concerns that sugar was harmful. Publishing a study in a prominent journal was a powerful tool for shaping scientific recommendations, and, unfortunately, medicine.

Another detriment to a healthy lifestyle was delivered in 1977 when the Select Committee on Nutrition and Human Needs released its *Dietary Goals for the United States*. The recommendations in this report led to the American Society for Clinical Nutrition's food pyramid. Fats were in the smallest triangle at the top with daily servings listed as "sparingly." Milk, cheese, and butter along with meat, fish, and eggs were the next smallest sections at 2-3 servings daily, followed by fruits and vegetables. The largest section at the bottom was 6-11 daily servings of bread, cereal, rice, and pasta. The largest section of the food pyramid was filled with "fake foods" that weren't even available in our ancestral diet. To make things worse, it included recommendations to replace saturated fat with industrialized vegetable and seed oils, which increased Omega-6 fats in the diet and decreased healthy Omega-3 fats. Instead, the recommendation was to take a fish oil supplement to replace healthy foods. The modern American diet contains an Omega-6 to Omega-3 ratio of 10:1 and sometimes as high as 30:1. Our ancestors had a diet with a ratio closer to 2:1. For optimal health, I recommend a ratio of about 4:1.

Within five years of the pyramid's widespread adoption, global rates of diabetes, obesity, and heart disease exploded. This was all driven by an increase in visceral fat, poor mitochondrial health, and a thick coat of inflammation. Anything boxed or bagged in the grocery store is likely to include canola, soybean, sunflower, or other easily oxidized seed oils. These oils date back to the early 1900s when soap makers discovered they could make a solid fat from a liquid, which contributed to the soap's lather and conditioning qualities. Then in 1910, a partially hydrogenated plant fat called Crisco® was released to the masses, which was supposed to replace butter and lard. The problem isn't with the plant fat itself but with the process by which it's made. When seed oil is exposed to heat, light, and oxygen, it oxidizes, which can release harmful compounds and toxic byproducts. To popularize seed oils and increase sales, the industry demonized animal fat (red meat, butter, milk, etc.) and succeeded. Even today, consumers believe the words "plant-based" on packages equate to being healthy.

Vegetable oil consumption is now at an all-time high, and

the amount of added flour, sugar, and seed oils in our food is astonishing. From 1800-2019, processed and ultra-processed food consumption went from <5% to more than 60%, the majority of those ingredients being wheat, rice, sugar, and vegetable oils. The solution is to get back to eating the way nature intended. The less processed your food, the better. Unfortunately, our government and medical system will not save you from the atrocity that has occurred over the last 100 years, which is a nation overfed and undernourished. Just look at the foods served to the most ill patients in hospitals—it is truly astonishing. You may save money now eating cheap, processed foods, but you will pay 10-fold back in health care expenses and time over your lifetime. Even the new *Dietary Guidelines for Americans* document released in 2020 encourages replacing butter with "nutrient-dense" vegetable oil—a toxic, whole food substitute. If the voice of this book is heard, I can only hope our government will recognize where they got it wrong. Society can no longer ignore a growing body of evidence for low carb, higher fat diets when it adopts the next set of guidelines in 2025. We must be louder than the special interest groups who continue to manipulate our diets and dismantle our health.

In 2019, the American Diabetes Association (ADA) released a consensus statement that lightly advocated for low carb and ketogenic diets. The ADA admitted that the amount of carbohydrate intake required for optimal health in humans is unknown. Currently, the ADA believes the minimum required daily carbs is 130g, determined in part by the brain's requirement for glucose, even though this energy requirement can be fulfilled by the body's metabolic processes, which include glycogenolysis, gluconeogenesis (via metabolism of the glycerol component of fat or gluconeogenic amino acids in protein), and/or ketogenesis in the setting of very low dietary carbohydrate intake. The ADA concluded that patients should be given individualized options for treatment of insulin resistance including low carb diets. These statements were then met with support from the American Heart Association in 2022, which stated that very low carbohydrate vs moderate carbohydrate diets yielded a greater decrease in hemoglobin A1c, greater weight loss, and use of fewer medications in individuals with insulin resistance and diabetes.

There is a prevalent insulin resistance problem in the U.S. and around the world. At the current trend, by 2050, 1 in 3 Americans will have Type 2 diabetes and many more will have pre-diabetes. If society continues to line the pockets of processed food manufacturers, they will continue to produce delicious, addictive foods full of sugar and toxic ingredients. They've mastered the perfect combination of unhealthy fats, sugars, and flavorings that are cheap, available, and keep people coming back for more. You need to make choices with your dollars that will elicit change. Hard to kill is a grass roots movement that starts with each one of us.

· · ·

Components of Food

What should you eat to be hard to kill? Eat whole foods that don't have a list of ingredients—they *are* the ingredient. A good rule of thumb is if it grew in the ground or had a mother, it's probably going to be better for your health. In this next section, I will discuss the basic food-related concepts and components that make up food.

Calorie: A calorie is a unit of energy. The body needs a certain number of energy units every day to operate its systems, such as breathing, digesting food, and regulating body temperature. Imagine your body is a bank account. The units of energy you consume (food) is income. The units of energy you expend doing activities (exercise) is debt. Early humans were designed to store or save energy units in case they had periods of famine—it was a mechanism to avoid starvation. So, income was more advantageous than debt.

Today, there is no lack of income. Thanks to refrigerators, freezers, and pantries, most people have plenty of food at all times. However, your body is still designed to save energy units, so when you have more income than debt, it can lead to poor health. The stored energy is not only subcutaneous fat but stored inside and around your organs in the form of visceral fat. The key is to maintain a balance. When it comes to the calories you consume, you don't want to be rich or poor. However, some studies show that caloric restriction may increase longevity over a lifetime. I mentioned earlier that I used to count calories. This practice might help you maintain a specific weight, but it won't help you function properly. Eating 2,000 calories a day of meat, fish, eggs, and vegetables is much better than eating 2,000 calories a day of donuts, candy, and potato chips. The quality of calories you consume is much more important than the quantity.

Macronutrients

The body requires large amounts of three primary macronutrients to function properly: fat, protein, and carbohydrates. Each macronutrient is measured in calories per gram—food labels list the total grams of each per serving. Proteins and carbohydrates are the least calorie-dense, and fat is the most calorie-dense. The following is an overview of each macronutrient.

Fat: Fat contains 9 calories per gram and serves as an energy source to keep the body warm, a substrate for hormone production, and aids in the absorption of fat-soluble vitamins. The fat you eat gets stored or used for energy. The body has an unlimited storage capacity for fat. The areas of your body where you can pinch fat is subcutaneous fat stored in your adipocytes (fat cells). Fat that is stored deeper, such as around and inside your organs, is called visceral fat. Visceral fat is very dangerous and a major indicator of metabolic disease. To delineate further, the body has both brown and white fat. Babies are born with more brown fat because it provides them with built-in heat (babies don't have the ability to shiver when cold). As you age and develop the ability to shiver, white fat replaces most brown fat and is stored in the thighs, hips, and stomach. Some fat—whether white or brown —is necessary for the endocrine system to help regulate metabolic homeostasis. Humans have an essential level of body fat.

There are three types of dietary fats: monounsaturated fats (MUFA), polyunsaturated fats (PUFA), and saturated fats. There's a misconception that all saturated fat is bad, and all unsaturated fat is good. MUFA have one double bond in the acid chain and the rest are single bonded carbon atoms. Many people think of olive oil, nuts, and avocados when it comes to this kind of fat. Red meat has almost as much MUFA as it does saturated fat. PUFAs have at least two double carbon bonds. The most common source of PUFAs in the American diet is not whole food sources. It is from plant seed oils like soybean and corn, which are unstable, easily oxidized, and pro-inflammatory. Saturated fat contains only single carbon bonds.

Food such as red meat is often vilified for its saturated fat content, but it actually contains almost as much monounsaturated fat in the form of oleic acid. Plant seed oil contains a higher proportion of polyunsaturated fat. In whole foods these polyunsaturated fats are ok, but as I've already discussed, vegetable oil is toxic to your body due to the fact that these fats are more easily oxidized, especially when heated, which drives inflammation and disease. A recent article in the *Journal of American College of Cardiology* reported that limiting foods rich in dietary saturated fats had no heart health benefits. The article stated, "Whole-fat dairy, unprocessed meat, eggs and dark chocolate are SFA [saturated fatty acid]-rich foods with a complex matrix that are not associated with increased risk of CVD [cardiovascular disease]. The totality of available evidence does not support further limiting the intake of such foods." In other words, don't blame the butter for what the bread does. When choosing which types of fat to eat, make sure you find a balance of healthy fats in all three categories and see how your body responds.

There is an essential intake of fat needed to survive. Fatty acids are essential for every cell membrane in the body and are also the precursor for your sex hormones like estrogen and testosterone. Yes, your hormones are made from cholesterol. To get the minimum of 3 grams of essential fatty acids, you need about 25-35% of calories coming from fat. This is why a low fat diet can be very detrimental to your health.

Protein: Protein contains 4 calories per gram and is another essential macronutrient. It acts as a building block for the body to produce muscle, bone, hair, skin, blood cells, and more. Scientists aren't sure, but the body may contain upwards of 20,000 different proteins. Protein also functions as a structural part of transporters, immune factors, hormones, enzymes, and neurotransmitters. Protein is composed of long chains of amino acids, or smaller building blocks. The body can't store amino acids so they must be ingested or made internally for health and survival. The following lists the nine essential amino acids that must be consumed through food:

Histidine: Red meat, beans, eggs, seafood, rice, buckwheat, bananas, citrus fruits

Valine: Red meat, chicken, pork, tuna, beans, nuts

Leucine: Red meat, lamb, poultry, cheese, pistachios, peanuts, sunflower seeds

Lysine: Red meat, cheese, fish, eggs, avocado, mango, beetroot, peppers

Methionine: Red meat, tuna, salmon, shrimp, lamb, soybeans

Isoleucine: Red meat, tuna, cod, haddock, yogurt, sunflower seeds, sesame seeds

Phenylalanine: Red meat, lamb, pork, poultry, cheese, eggs, yogurt, nuts

Threonine: Red meat, lamb, pork, cheese, almonds, pistachios

Tryptophan: Red meat, turkey, dark chocolate, milk, cheese, eggs, fish, chickpeas, nuts

To be considered a complete protein, a food must contain all 9 essential amino acids. Proteins come from either plants or animals, but the two sources are vastly different. Animal-based protein is high quality and nutrient dense, whereas to obtain a similar amount of protein from only plants, you'd have to consume much larger amounts, which also results in eating more carbohydrates. A varied diet with paired plant proteins throughout the day is also necessary to obtain all essential amino acids if you are eating a vegan, vegetarian, or plant-based diet. Animal foods like red meat and eggs are very nutrient dense and contain all nine essential amino acids.

The current recommended dietary allowance (RDA) for protein is far too low. At the current RDA of 0.8g/kg, a 200-pound person would get only 72g per day. This number is the bare minimum to simply stay alive. It's not what you want to eat if you want to be hard to kill. If you are active or aging, you need to eat much more than this. The amount of protein you eat should be based on your goals:

Minimum: 0.8/kg bodyweight

Sedentary: 1.2-1.4/kg bodyweight

Active muscle building: 1.6-2.2g/kg bodyweight

Aging adults, those with severe illness, or those in a deep caloric deficit may benefit from >2.2g/kg bodyweight

I personally aim for 2.2g/kg, which equates to 1 gram per pound of body weight. If you weigh 160 pounds, that is 160g of protein per day. Eating this amount of protein will ensure good leucine content, which drives muscle protein synthesis. It also helps with insulin signaling and your ability to burn fat. Once again, animal proteins are a great source of leucine as well as other essential amino acids like lysine and methionine.

Carbohydrates: Carbohydrates contain 4 calories per gram and are *non-essential* for human life. You could live entirely on fat and protein and never consume a single carbohydrate. Through a process called gluconeogenesis, the body can produce essential amounts of carbohydrates from protein and fat stores. Does this mean you shouldn't ever eat carbs? Not at all. Everyone is unique and you must determine what your body needs for optimal health. However, the body can only store up to 2,000 calories of carbs in the form of glycogen. It's similar to having a wallet that can only hold up to $2,000 cash. If you spend some of that cash, you have room to put more money in your wallet, but only until it reaches $2,000 again. Athletes often "carb load" prior to competing to ensure they have a wallet full of cash to spend during competition.

Unfortunately, most people keep their carb wallet full without ever spending any of it, which ultimately slows them down and they lose the health race. Carbohydrates are not inherently evil, but the overconsumption of them will be detrimental to you. Current recommendations of 45-65% carbs in the diet is too much for our sedentary society. It is also mathematically impossible to get all the essential nutrients and minerals you need in a calorically appropriate diet eating that many carbs.

Micronutrients

In addition to macronutrients, food contains micronutrients such as vitamins and minerals. These smaller layers, in addition to the larger building blocks and energy units, must all be consumed and don't occur naturally in the body. That's why eating whole food is so vital for optimal health. Most processed foods are energy dense in calories from carbs and fat and devoid of nutrients unless fortified.

Metabolic Health: According to the 2018 *National Health and Nutrition Examination Survey* published by the Centers for Disease Control and Prevention (CDC), 88% of Americans have abnormal metabolic markers: fasting blood glucose, triglycerides, high density lipoprotein cholesterol, blood pressure, and waist circumference.

Each of these markers should be within normal range without the use of medication to be considered metabolically healthy. Currently, approximately 422 million people across the world live with Type 2 diabetes and many more million live with pre-diabetes and insulin resistance, which leads to Type 2 diabetes if there is no intervention. The worst part is most of them don't even realize they have it. I was one of those people, walking around with pre-diabetes without knowing it.

. . .

The Metabolic Machine

According to the World Health Organization (WHO), since 1975 obesity around the world has tripled with more than 1.9 billion adults overweight—and that doesn't include children. During the first year of the pandemic, Type 2 diabetes rose more than 182%. Obesity and insulin resistance are key drivers of heart disease, which is the leading cause of death in Americans, followed by cancer. The solution is to teach your body how to become a metabolic machine, which means emptying its carbohydrate tank so your body can tap into its fat stores. This means eliminating flours, added sugar, and toxic seed oils, and increasing your consumption of protein and fat. The result will be a period of ketogenic adaptation.

Limiting carbohydrates to a specific threshold lowers the hormone insulin and forces your body to rely on fat as an energy substrate, which can promote weight loss if calories are controlled. First, you must burn through your glycogen (stored carbs in the liver). As this happens, your body secretes a counter regulatory hormone called glucagon. This stimulates gluconeogenesis—a process in which your body makes its own glucose from lactic acid, glycerol, and the amino acids alanine and glutamine. During this process, ketogenesis begins.

Ketones are derived from fat—whether from body or

dietary fat. Ketone bodies do so much more than just provide an energy substrate. They also work as cellular signaling molecules that serve as an efficient source of fuel, boost the immune system, and reduce inflammation. Your glucose levels are tightly regulated in the body and glucose is always present. The goal is to teach your body metabolic flexibility. This will allow your body to use both glucose and fat efficiently as energy substrates. By reducing the burden of high glucose and high insulin, your body can learn to burn fat again instead of storing it. It's normal for people to go in and out of ketosis. Our ancestors did it, pregnant women do it, and newborn babies do it. It's a part of our physiology that we have ignored. Most people override this innate process by adopting years and years of poor eating habits and consuming too many processed carbohydrates.

It's easy to reprogram your body and only takes about 2-4 days eating a low carb diet for your body to achieve a state of ketosis. During periods of fasting or carbohydrate restriction, the body suppresses insulin. Insulin is a hormone that is secreted in response to dietary carbohydrates or some proteins. With suppression of insulin and depletion of glycogen (the $2,000 wallet analogy) the body accelerates oxidation of fat (fatty acids) to produce these ketones. The ketogenic (keto) diet is the only diet that has a biomarker. You can test your ketone level at any time through blood, breath, or urine to measure your ketone level. No other diet has this capability. The ketogenic diet was originally researched as a diet to prevent seizures in epileptic children. The traditional ketogenic diet used a ratio of around 4:1 fat to protein + carbohydrates. Most people don't need this level of therapeutic ketosis and would benefit from a 1:1 ratio, modified low-carb diet, or even a low glycemic index diet.

The ketogenic diet is contraindicated in certain individuals. Those with pancreatitis, liver failure, disorders of fat metabolism, primary carnitine deficiency, porphyrias, carnitine palmitoyltransferase deficiency, carnitine translocase deficiency or pyruvate kinase deficiency should work directly with a provider for nutritional therapy. Additionally, anyone using medication, especially for diabetes or high blood pressure, may need rapid reduction in medication and should be monitored closely. Become educated about what is going on inside your body, and know your numbers.

The graphs on the following pages illustrate these diets:

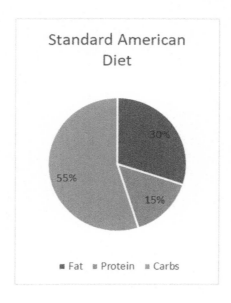

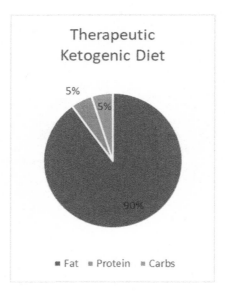

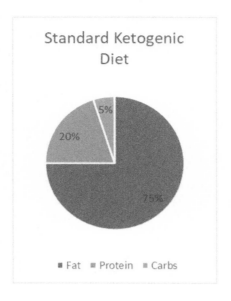

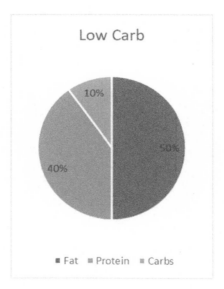

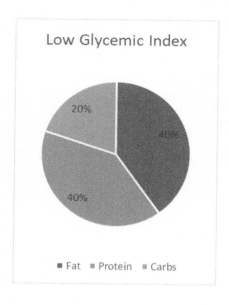

For most people, protein should be prioritized in the diet. Fat should fill out the meals and carbohydrates should be earned based on activity and body composition. When you join the Hard to Kill Academy (found online), I'll give you step-by-step instructions to achieve ketosis and ketogenic adaptation. A standard keto diet comprises 75-80% fat calories, 15-20% protein calories, and 5-10% carbohydrate calories. Not all low carbohydrate diets are equal and everything must be in the context of your goals. There are variations of the keto diet, such as the carnivore diet, which excludes all plants. Autoimmune diseases and gut issues often improve when excluding plants for a period of time because of some defense mechanisms found in plants like lectins, oxalates, and phytic acid. For some people, fibrous plants are ok and can help satiety, slow digestion, and nourish the gut microbiome. In my opinion outside of personal, ethical beliefs, an animal-based diet provides the most bioavailable protein and nutrients to nourish your body. Everyone will respond differently to different carb thresholds, but I want you to understand it is a spectrum of dietary approaches from therapeutic ketosis, to low carb, to a low glycemic index. Feel free to experiment so you can decide how you feel and function best.

Once you've repaired the metabolic damage and insulin resistance from your previous diet, then you might be able to add some whole food carbohydrates back into it. Carbohydrates are not the devil; overconsumption of processed carbohydrates is. Similarly, fat is good for you, but overconsumption of low quality, processed fat will lead to poor metabolic health and disease. Protein is the key—it has a satiating effect to help control hunger and cravings and has its own thermogenic effect on the body, which boosts metabolic burn. The goal of the Hard to Kill eating plan is to eat adequate protein and control your energy calories from fat and carbohydrates. Remember, eat only whole foods that were grown in the earth or once had a mother. This type of diet will support lean body mass, bones, and connective tissue, making you hard to kill.

There will always be exceptions to the rule. We all know someone who practiced an unhealthy lifestyle but lived well into old age. Winston Churchill smoked, drank, and lived a happy obese life until the age of 90. I don't know how much time you or I have left, but I do know we have control over the time we do have. You especially have control over what you eat, so if you want to be hard to kill, eat a nutrient-dense, whole food diet with plenty of fat and protein. Doctors are also finding a lot of genetic variation in how people respond to these different dietary approaches. I've included a sample list of which foods to eat and not to eat on the Hard to Kill plan. This list is not exhaustive but should give you a general idea and starting point. I've also included some examples in a sample menu to show you the different levels of carbohydrate intake I have tried. Bon appétit!

Recommended Hard to Kill Foods

Protein:
- Seafood including fatty fish
- Ruminant animals (beef, lamb, elk, deer, buffalo)
- Eggs
- Poultry (chicken, turkey, duck, etc.)
- Non-ruminant animals (pork, boar, rabbit, kangaroo)

Fats:
- Animal fats
- Butter and dairy

- Ghee
- Tallow
- Coconut oil
- Olive oil
- Avocado oil
- MCT oil
- Nuts/seeds
- Other great fats—avocados, coconut, olives, cacao butter

Low carb/Ketogenic Fruits and Vegetables:
- Sweet potato
- Butternut squash
- Spaghetti squash
- Parsnips
- Carrots
- Purple potato
- Pumpkin
- Apples
- Bananas
- Pears
- Oranges
- Blackberries
- Blueberries
- Raspberries
- Strawberries
- Broccoli

- Kale
- Peppers
- Onions
- Tomatoes
- Yams
- Turnips
- Avocados

Moderate carb/Paleo Fruits and Vegetables:
- Sweet potatoes
- Butternut squash
- Spaghetti squash
- Parsnips
- Carrots
- Purple potatoes
- Pumpkin
- Apples
- Bananas
- Pears
- Oranges
- Blackberries
- Blueberries
- Strawberries
- Broccoli
- Kale
- Peppers

- Onions
- Tomatoes
- Yams
- Turnips
- Avocados

Hard to Kill Foods to Avoid

- Refined grains (wheat, barley, rolled oats, rice, corn meal)
- Breads made with refined grains
- Pasta made with refined grains
- Cookies, crackers, cakes, or similar
- Added sugars (agave nectar, high fructose corn syrup, cane sugar, maple syrup, refined honey)
- Vegetable oil and seed oils (canola, corn, grapeseed, cottonseed, peanut, sesame, safflower)
- Alcohol
- Soft drinks and juices
- Margarines or plant butters
- Plant milks (almond, oat, etc.)
- Packaged foods

Sample Menus

Ketogenic Menu:

Meal 1: 3 pastured eggs and ½ avocado

Meal 2: 10-oz. grass-fed beef burger, 1 cup roasted broccoli, 10 macadamia nuts

Meal 3: 8-oz. wild-caught salmon, 1 cup shaved or roasted Brussels sprouts

Macros: 1761 calories, Protein 127g (29%), Fat 130g (65%), Carbs 28g (6%)

Ketogenic Carnivore Menu:

Meal 1: 4 pastured eggs, 1 Tbsp ghee

Meal 2: 8-oz. chicken breast, 1-oz. gouda cheese

Meal 3: 8-oz. ribeye steak, 1 Tbsp salmon roe, 4-oz wild-caught shrimp

Macros: 1677 calories, Protein 152g (40%), Fat 102g (60%), Carbs 3g (0%)

Low carb Menu:

Meal 1: 3 pastured eggs, 1 medium apple, ½ avocado

Meal 2: 8-oz. ground beef, ¾ cup cubed sweet potato, 1 cup cucumber salad

Meal 3: 8-oz. grilled wild-caught salmon with 1 Tbsp. avocado oil and lemon pepper, ½ cup blueberries, 1 cup roasted broccoli, 10 macadamia nuts

Macros: 1746 calories, Protein 124g (28%), Fat 109g (55%), Carbs 76g (17%)

• • •

Each menu includes at least 40g of protein, three times per day. This helps promote satiety, which reduces the desire for processed carbohydrates. When transitioning to a low-carb diet, be careful not to over consume nuts and cheeses or add processed low-carb foods. Focus on fatty, nutrient-dense animal food. Moderate fat to your energy needs and keep carbs at your personal threshold to ensure success.

Fasting and Meal Frequency

Growing up as an athlete, I was told to eat multiple times per day. Most body-builders and athletes use this approach to maximize muscle protein synthesis. The theory is that this keeps the metabolism running and helps you lose fat and retain lean body mass. However, multiple studies show this does not appear to significantly affect body composition or boost metabolism. What you consume in a 24 hour period matters more. As a mom and busy professional, eating six times per day is not feasible. When I adopted a low carb lifestyle, I also incorporated fasting, or intermittent eating. Most days I break my fast around noon. Breakfast literally means to break your fast and can be done at any hour, not just when you wake up. It is very important when you break a fast that the meal contains 30-50g of high quality protein.

Intermittent fasting, or time-restricted feeding, involves choosing a window of time to eat your calories for the day. The most popular method is a 16:8 method—you fast for 16 hours and then eat all your meals in an 8 hour window. You could make your eating window smaller but you risk under nourishment and a lack of adequate protein. It's important to pick the same window every day. Due to biological circadian clocks, your body anticipates meals even before that first bite. Your body likes the routine.

You can also perform alternate day fasting. This involves eating breakfast, lunch, and dinner one day and then only dinner the following day—essentially 24 hours between your dinners. Alternate day fasting has been shown to be an effective strategy at reducing fasting glucose and fasting insulin levels even when consuming larger amounts of carbohydrates. Fasting is just a tool and is not required. When incorporated appropriately, restricting how often you eat helps elevate blood ketone levels and increase reliance on fat as a fuel source.

Extended fasting is when you don't eat for more than 24 hours. Fasting is a form of hormetic stress. Just like sprinting, saunas, and ice baths, it too can be overdone and can hinder your progress. Fasting can increase stress hormones like cortisol and norepinephrine. It also helps stimulate autophagy, as does exercise. Autophagy constantly occurs in your body and means "eating yourself". It's a process by which the body cleans up dead and damaged cells.

Longevity researchers have studied the effects of fasting and fasting mimicking diets like the ketogenic diet with promising results. Some people perform these extended fasts just a few times per year. They are also used in religion like the ramadan fast. It is theorized that extended fasts purge the body of damaged cells such as cancer cells. If you perform fasting you may want to consider use of water and electrolytes. If you don't consume them, that is considered "dry fasting" and can be dangerous if not monitored properly or if done for too long.

Whether or not you fast is up to you. Emerging evidence shows other benefits, especially to the immune system and an overall reduction in inflammation. A study released in the summer of 2022 showed that people who intermittently fasted experienced fewer severe complications from COVID-19. This all goes back to not overconsuming and ensuring you eat in moderation. Find what works best for you.

Animal-based Diets

I've highlighted how our ancestors thrived on animal foods and smaller amounts of plants. I fear that the political movement of "plant-based diets" will further push people into eating highly processed, carbohydrate-dense foods. If you want to be hard to kill, animal foods contain many things that you can't find in plants. These include vitamin B12, creatine, carnosine, vitamin D3, Docosahexaenoic acid (DHA), heme iron, and taurine. Creatine is one of the most studied supplements in the exercise world. Increasing creatine improves athletic performance, increases muscle mass, and improves brain function. Why would you want to avoid that?

As an OBGYN, I constantly think about my pregnant patients and the nutrients required to build a human. These nutrients come from animal foods such as eggs, organ meats, beef, fish, dairy, and bone broth. I advise against plant-based, vegetarian, or vegan diets for this reason. Without a lot of titration and supplementation, you would be deficient in Vitamin B12, iron, DHA, zinc, Vitamin K2, preformed vitamin A, choline, and glycine. Red meat in particular has been politicized to an extreme. Americans have been told red meat is bad for you. Its consumption peaked in 1971 and has tumbled ever since, yet metabolic disease continues to rise. Humans have been eating meat for 2.5 millions years. It is a true super-food that will make you hard to kill. We are being mislead and distracted by the emotions of eating animals. Anthropologists believe humans developed large, intelligent brains by eating red meat. There is no strong evidence that meat is dangerous. Eat meat, and stay hard to kill.

Chapter 4
Pillar 2: Movement

Fitness Failure
    Society's reliance on convenience has made people lazy. Everyone is guilty of driving too much, taking time to find the closest parking space, using elevators and escalators instead of stairs, and even standing on the moving walkway at the airport. Going to the gym is only reserved for "spare time," and once there, many people do nothing other than cardio. It's no wonder people are the unhealthiest they've ever been.

    The fitness industry is extremely profitable because people waste so much of their money on it. Gyms rely on the fact that many of its members either don't show up or don't achieve sustainable results. Social media has exacerbated the problem by flooding news feeds with the latest workout and diet fads: 30 days to 6-pack abs, 10-day celery juice cleanse, or 8 weeks to get shredded. Even I'm guilty of purchasing online workouts that I only used once or twice.

The relapse rate for diets and workouts is high, and studies estimate the failure rate of the fitness industry to be 92%. Imagine if you had failed in school 92% of the time! Additionally, the benefit you gain from cardio exercise is lost once you stop. Even after I trained and ran the half marathon to "get healthy," I still developed pre-diabetes because of my poor diet. You can't out-cardio bad nutrition habits, which is why nutrition is the first pillar of the Hard to Kill plan. Plain and simple, having muscle mass will make you hard to kill.

Body Composition

To have a more informed discussion about health, it's important to understand body composition. A body composition test estimates how much fat and lean body mass you have. Some techniques can also detect how much fat you have that is subcutaneous (under the skin) and visceral (around the organs). A regular scale like one you may have at home doesn't differentiate between fat and muscle. Plus, weight can fluctuate by the day and even by the hour, especially for women, depending on hydration, digestion, and the menstrual cycle. My preferred way to measure body composition is through a DEXA (Dual Energy X-ray Absorptiometry) scan, but you can also use an MRI, CT scan, BOD POD®, bioelectrical impedance scale, under water weighing, calipers, or even a flexible tape measure with an online calculator. Even without a calculation most men should have a waist circumference less than 40 inches and women less than 35 inches for good health. Or you can calculate a waist to hip ratio. For women it should be <0.7 and for men <0.85. The waist to hip ratio correlates with visceral fat. Women who have a waist to hip ratio over 0.85 have three times the risk of developing coronary heart disease. Just choose a method that's readily available so you can have consistent data over time and track your progress.

WOMEN	
Classification	Body Fat Percentage
Obese	32% or more
Acceptable	25-31%
Fitness	21-24%
Athlete	14-20%
Essential Body Fat	10-13%

MEN	
Classification	Body Fat Percentage
Obese	25% or more
Acceptable	18-25%
Fitness	14-17%
Athlete	6-13%
Essential Body Fat	2-5%

In addition to measuring your body fat and lean body mass, its important to know how much visceral fat you have. The fat you can pinch on your body is called subcutaneous fat and lies underneath the skin. Visceral fat is deep inside your belly and inside and around your organs. Its what gives people more of an "apple" shape appearance and it's the reason why waist circumference is a good indicator that you may have too much. Visceral fat is linked directly with heart disease, diabetes, cancer, stroke, and other metabolic diseases. The more visceral fat you have and the longer you have it create more risk. This is why your body weight and BMI can be misleading—they don't measure visceral fat.

Methods to measure visceral fat include a DEXA scan, CT, and MRI. MRI would be best as it avoids any use of radiation. In some cities you can pay cash to get an MRI with an order from your doctor. That option is available where I live for about $450. The more available option is a DEXA scan and costs about $100 where I live. The DEXA scan will measure your Visceral Fat Area (VFA). An ideal VFA score for women is <85 and <100 for men. The other component to assess is the visceral to subcutaneous fat (VSR) ratio. For men the VSR should be less than 1 and for women less than 0.5. Anything above this threshold is highly predictive of insulin resistance, diabetes, and metabolic disease.

DEXA Measurements of Visceral Fat

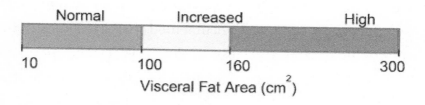

MRI Measurements of Visceral Fat

Visceral Fat Mass Percentile by Age (Female)

	0% - 20%	20% - 40%	40% - 60%	60% - 80%	> 80%
20-29	< 0.03 lbs	0.03 lbs – 0.17 lbs	0.17 lbs – 0.35 lbs	0.35 lbs – 0.70 lbs	> 0.7 lbs
30-39	< 0.09 lbs	0.09 lbs – 0.26 lbs	0.26 lbs – 0.51 lbs	0.51 lbs – 1.02 lbs	> 1.02 lbs
40-49	< 0.17 lbs	0.17 lbs – 0.42 lbs	0.42 lbs – 0.80 lbs	0.80 lbs – 1.51 lbs	> 1.51 lbs
50-59	< 0.27 lbs	0.27 lbs – 0.60 lbs	0.60 lbs – 1.07 lbs	1.07 lbs – 1.88 lbs	> 1.88 lbs
60+	< 0.52 lbs	0.52 lbs – 1.01 lbs	1.01 lbs – 1.58 lbs	1.58 lbs – 2.48 lbs	> 2.48 lbs

Visceral Fat Mass Percentile by Age (Male)

	0% - 20%	20% - 40%	40% - 60%	60% - 80%	> 80%
20-29	< 0.18 lbs	0.18 lbs – 0.40 lbs	0.40 lbs – 0.66 lbs	0.66 lbs – 1.11 lbs	> 1.11 lbs
30-39	< 0.37 lbs	0.37 lbs – 0.72 lbs	0.72 lbs – 1.20 lbs	1.20 lbs – 2.05 lbs	> 2.05 lbs
40-49	< 0.64 lbs	0.64 lbs – 1.19 lbs	1.19 lbs – 1.97 lbs	1.97 lbs – 3.14 lbs	> 3.14 lbs
50-59	< 0.87 lbs	0.87 lbs – 1.58 lbs	1.58 lbs – 2.43 lbs	2.43 lbs – 3.72 lbs	> 3.72 lbs
60+	< 1.19 lbs	1.19 lbs – 2.07 lbs	2.07 lbs – 3.18 lbs	3.18 lbs – 4.56 lbs	> 4.56 lbs

Correct Movement Matters

All movement is good movement, but movement that improves muscle mass will leverage your metabolic health and make you harder to kill. Remember, most people are not "over fat" they are "under muscled". You need to worry more about how much weight you can lift and less about how much you weigh. It's been well-documented that strength training reduces the risk of all causes of death. Weight lifting is the best bio-hack available. People who have more physical strength are less likely to develop cardiovascular disease, diabetes, cancer, or any other condition that can cause an early death. A Harvard University study followed 1,100 healthy men with an average age of 40 and had them perform as many push-ups as they could in one minute. Ten years later, they found that the men who performed 40 or more push-ups were 96% less likely to develop cardiovascular disease than the men who performed 10 or fewer push-ups.

Another simple test you can do at home is the chair test. Sit down in a chair without using your arms or hands and do the same while standing back up. It's a simple test that easily assesses flexibility, balance, motor coordination, and strength in the large muscle groups. According to research, people middle-aged and the elderly who need to put their hands on their knees in order to sit down and stand up are seven times more likely to die within six years.

A variation of the chair test can assess your current strength level. Perform the chair test 10 times and record how long it takes you to complete it (recommended times are below). The chair test and the push-up metric aren't about impressing your friends or family. They are a guide for thriving given your time on earth. I love to hike, swim in the ocean, and vacation with my family, and I want to continue to enjoy those activities as I become older. Someday I also want to be able to get down on the floor and play with my grandkids as well as to live independently. Find out what brings you joy in life and make sure you're able to do those activities until the end.

. . .

Chair Test (sitting and standing 10 times unassisted):

Men's Expected Times	Women's Expected Times
Under 35 Years: 10 Seconds	Under 35 Years: 12 Seconds
35-55 Years: 13 Seconds	35-55 Years: 15 Seconds
Over 55 Years: 18 Seconds	Over 55 Years: 19 Seconds

Measurements of Movement

Going back to the analogy that your body is like a bank account and you need to balance your income and spending, there are four ways you can spend, or burn energy calories:

BMR—Basal Metabolic Rate (includes resting metabolic rate or expenditure): The calories you burn while the body performs basic physiologic functions, as well as the calories burned while resting or sleeping. This accounts for roughly 70% of the calories you use.

NEAT—Non-Exercise Activity Thermogenesis: the calories you burn for everything you do that is not sleeping, eating, or purposeful exercise. This includes activities such as working at your desk, taking the stairs, gardening, or cooking.

EAT—Exercise Activity Thermogenesis: The calories you burn during purposeful exercise.

TEF—Thermic Effect of Food: The calories you burn to digest your food after you eat.

Some people may think they can't control their BMR, but

that's not true. The more muscle you have, the more calories you'll burn while resting. Getting adequate sleep is also critical for your BMR, and I'll address sleep in the next chapter.

You've probably heard the recommendation to get at least 10,000 steps every day. These steps only apply to NEAT calories, such as walking from your car into work, taking stairs instead of an elevator, or walking to the mailbox. Continuing to find ways to increase your NEAT calories outside of purposeful exercise every day is an important component of overall movement.

I spent a lot of time discussing nutrition in the last chapter. Can you guess which foods have the highest thermic effect, or TEF? It's whole foods, especially proteins such as lean red meat, fish, chicken, and eggs. Eating these types of food will increase the calories your body burns during digestion.

The final method, EAT, which is purposeful exercise, is the focus of the rest of this chapter. Though walking and other forms of cardio have value, they don't help build muscle. Prolonged cardio sessions on a treadmill or elliptical machine might actually promote muscle breakdown and hinder your ability to burn fat. If cardio sessions are too long, it can increase your cortisol, putting your muscle mass at risk and hindering fat loss. Compare the body composition of a marathon runner to a sprinter. Most marathon runners have significantly less lean muscle mass than sprinters.

Professional sprinters only train for about 12 minutes per day. Longer doesn't mean better results. Training needs to be efficient and effective at providing a stimulus, and no more.

If your goal is to burn body fat, then I recommend high-intensity interval training (HIIT), such as sprinting. The best part is that you only need to do it for minutes to get maximum benefit. This is good news for busy professionals or moms like me who have a hard time finding more than 30 minutes to work out. HIIT training generally means you are working at a level that requires about 80-100% of your max heart rate. Your maximum heart rate can be estimated by taking 220 minus your age in years. This is opposed to lower intensity, which can be done for much longer and at a much lower heart rate, about 50-70% of your max heart rate.

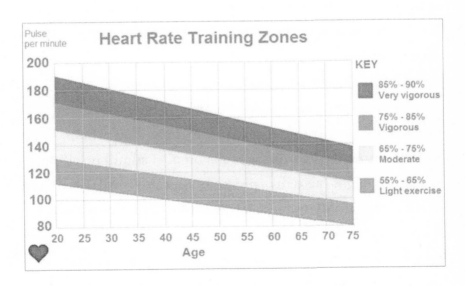

Traditionally, fitness instructors tell you to do low

intensity, steady-state cardio to burn fat. It is all a difference of immediate fuel source, but HIIT such as sprinting is a fantastic way to empty your glucose wallet. Sprint interval training has been studied in women and men of all ages as well as people with disabilities and pre- and post-menopausal women, all with the same favorable results. It increases total lean body mass, decreases fat mass, improves aerobic capacity, and improves biomarkers of metabolic health. If you're already familiar with HIIT, sprint interval training is like HIIT on steroids. Here is a sample sprint interval training session:

1. Sprint on a treadmill or pedal on a bike as fast as you can for 30 seconds at maximum effort
2. Slow down to a jog, walk, or slow pedal for 2 minutes
3. Repeat 8 times. Do this 3-4 days per week

It really can be any movement, done at absolute maximum effort. This means you can do it anywhere in the world, at any time, with no equipment except a timer, which can be found on your phone.

If you aren't comfortable with sprinting, then focus on lower intensity, steady-state exercise. There is still good evidence that 180-200 minutes per week of moderate activity reduces all-cause mortality and reduces cardiovascular disease. In other words, just move!

. . .

Building Muscle

Now that you understand the different types of movement for burning calories, I'll discuss moving to build muscle. As you age, you naturally lose muscle mass, which is called age-related sarcopenia and happens in the absence of disease. Sarcopenia reduces your ability to perform activities of daily living and contributes to a loss of mobility and independence. It makes you frail and more likely to suffer a fall, which greatly increases your risk of disease and death. In other words, sarcopenia makes you easy to kill, which is why muscle is considered an organ of longevity.

It's important to build muscle strength as early as possible. Age-related sarcopenia begins in your 40s and accelerates in your 70s. After age 50, muscle mass decreases at an annual rate of 1-2%. Between ages 50-60 it decreases by another 1.5% per year, and then 3% every year after that. It's caused by a conversion from fast muscle twitch fibers into slow muscle twitch fibers, so you don't have as much strength to perform activities of daily living. This cascades into other pathological changes such as inflammation, loss of testosterone (needed to build muscle), and overall poor metabolic health. This is why weight and body mass index (BMI) alone aren't good markers of health. Only body composition tells the whole story, and, unfortunately, that story is that society is not only "over fat" but "under muscled" once again. Frailty and age-related sarcopenia are one of the greatest threats to your health.

Contrary to popular belief, skin isn't the largest organ, muscle is. Skin has greater surface area, but pound for pound, muscle is the winner. Skin is only about 5% of total body mass, whereas muscle can be 30-70%, depending on sex and body composition. Many people know their body fat percentage, but do you know your lean muscle mass percentage? Neither fat nor muscle are inert. Fat and muscle both act as part of the endocrine system, sending messages to other organs. Muscle contracts to move your skeleton, and when you move or lift heavy loads, it releases chemical messengers called myokines, which produce many effects, one of those being anti-inflammatory effects.

Muscle also helps with fat oxidation as well as glucose and protein metabolism. Muscles store the little building blocks—amino acids—discussed in the nutrition chapter. These layers of building blocks go through cycles of breaking down and rebuilding, which is called muscle protein synthesis. Although nutrition is a key component to muscle protein synthesis, lifting weighted objects will send your muscles a message that you still need them. A combination of eating adequate protein and lifting is necessary to support your muscles.

As you age, you develop anabolic resistance. This means the anabolic stimulus becomes diminished and muscle protein synthesis suffers. This actually happens any time in your life when you become inactive, sit in a chair for long periods, or are bed ridden. Disuse will cause loss. The previous chapter discussed the importance of protein. Due to anabolic resistance as you age you also need more protein to overcome these changes.

Therapeutic Ketosis

You can build muscle by consuming carbohydrates, but over time, age and insulin resistance will start decreasing your lean body mass. Another strategy to prevent age-related muscle loss is therapeutic ketosis. Ketones are produced in the liver as a byproduct of broken-down fat cells. There is evidence that ketones can help maintain lean muscle mass even during weight loss, which is ideal when trying to lose a large amount of weight. If a patient needs to lose 100 pounds, they want that to be 100 pounds of fat and not muscle. I lost a considerable amount of body fat while increasing my lean body mass.

In March of 2018, I weighed 173 pounds with 71.9 pounds of lean body mass and 45.9 pounds of fat mass, giving me a body fat percentage of 26.4% (left photo). Fast forward one year to March of 2019, I weighed 163.7 pounds with 79.1 pounds of lean body mass and 25.2 pounds of fat mass, giving me a body fat percentage of 15.4% (right photo). Most people would be disappointed if they only lost 10 pounds in a year with the amount of dieting and weight lifting I did. Yet when you break down these numbers, I lost just over 20 pounds of pure body fat and gained 7.2 pounds of muscle, all while eating a carnivore-ketogenic diet in a caloric deficit.

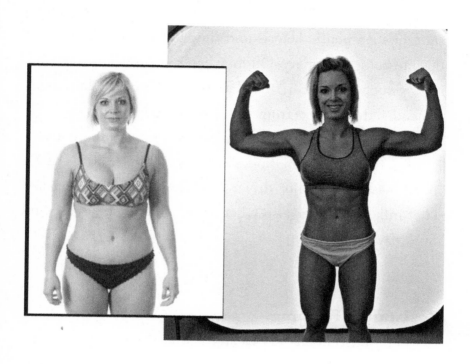

Ketogenic therapy is being studied for things like cancer cachexia and age-related sarcopenia. Ketones are thought to be anti-catabolic. This means they are protecting you from breaking down your own muscle tissue for fuel. Ketones preserve oxidative muscle fibers and improve both mitochondrial and antioxidant capacity within muscle. This simply means there is less protein turnover and better maintenance of lean muscle mass over time.

Two metabolic processes are constantly trying to

maintain a balance in your body: catabolism—breaking down muscle—and anabolism—building it back up. Therapeutic ketosis can help maintain this balance. There are many instances of bedridden hospital patients who are put into a state of therapeutic ketosis and they don't lose muscle mass despite being stationary. Often, when someone has a terminal illness such as cancer, the disease itself doesn't kill them. Instead, they die from metabolic complications that accompany the illness. Another way to protect muscle tissue is to reduce inflammation. Ketones inhibit the NLRP3 inflammasome, a major driver of inflammation in the body. That inflammation is also what drives metabolic disease and muscle wasting.

Resistance Training

The nutrition chapter established the type of food to eat and the percentage of macronutrients to consume in a day. This chapter determined that sprint interval training is the optimal way to burn fat. Next is to discuss how to build muscle so that you become stronger, leaner, and harder to kill. There is a misconception that having large muscles automatically means you're strong and having smaller muscles means you're weak. Everyone is born with a pre-set genetic potential with regard to physical form. Optimizing your diet, hormones, sleep, and exercise can be synergistic to that genetic makeup. As an undergraduate in exercise science, I studied research about how to encourage muscle adaptation so it's forced to grow. There are two ways that muscle can build and grow: hypertrophy, which is the process of existing muscle cells (fibers) becoming larger, and hyperplasia, which is an increase in the number of muscle fibers. To stimulate muscle growth, you have to create tension and load, which can be done using free weights, barbells, kettlebells, machines, resistance bands, or even body weight. Resistance training is a purposeful stress. When you perform resistance training, you release growth hormone, testosterone, myokines, and more. You also increase blood flow and nutrients to the muscle. Regardless of what kind of weight you use, there are three components needed for muscle growth:

1. *Volume:* The number of sets or repetitions combined with the actual weight you move. By progressively increasing volume, you increase the load on the muscle. For example, you can lift 20 pounds and then increase to 30 pounds, or you can lift 20 pounds for more repetitions. To increase volume you increase either reps, sets, weight or all of them. Volume creates time under tension for the muscle.

2. *Rest:* To build muscle, you must give it appropriate rest. Not too much time, but enough to recover and go again.

3. *Contraction:* There are two types of muscle contractions: concentric, which is the muscle shortening, and eccentric, which is the muscle lengthening. When you curl your arm during a bicep curl, the muscle shortens. When you straighten your arm, the muscle lengthens. Focus on squeezing your muscle during the concentric phase followed by a slow, controlled eccentric phase. Weight lifting should be purposeful and you need to always be mentally engaged. You're not actually training just your muscles; you're training your central nervous system, too, by controlling how you move that weight in space.

You can lift weights in as little as 20 minutes a day if you are efficient. For me, it shouldn't take more than 45-60 minutes. Resistance training can be performed as a full body workout or split into upper/lower or different body parts. There are many excellent programs available these days, or you can find workouts in The Hard to Kill Academy online. Make sure you always train opposing muscle groups so you don't create imbalances within the body. For example, if you train biceps, you want to train the opposing muscle, the triceps.

Resistance training also encourages bone mass growth, which helps prevent osteoporosis. Bone tissue, just like muscle, requires the attention of all five pillars of health. Peak bone mass occurs between the ages of 9-18. Bone loss begins in your 60s and rapidly declines in your 70s. Men tend to have larger statures than women and have more testosterone, so they lose less bone mass. Men have an annual bone loss rate of .82% per year. Women have an annual bone loss rate of .96% per year and are four times more likely to develop osteopenia and osteoporosis after age 50 due to decreases in mostly estrogen and some testosterone after menopause. Even though men lose less bone mass, they have more resulting complications. In the first year after sustaining a hip fracture, men have a 31% mortality rate and women have a 17% mortality rate. In other words, your risk of death triples the year after a hip fracture. Falls are the top cause of injury and injury-related death in people older than 65. If you do not want to lose your independence, you need to become strong and active right now. There is a direct correlation between losing lean muscle mass and losing bone mass. The good news is that you can protect your bones—and muscles—through the nutrition and resistance training outlined in this chapter.

Strength is Human

Being healthy isn't about looking strong. Ask your family and friends to perform the chair test. I'm sure some of them may "look" like they should easily be able to do it, but can they? I've discussed the body image issues I had for much of my life. Embracing my physical strength as a woman has never been easy for me, even as an athlete. Society told me time and time again that muscles equal masculinity and you can't be strong, feminine, and beautiful. It's time to eliminate this notion. As a mom of three girls, every day I strive to model the importance of physical strength as a hard to kill trait.

Female athletes actually have higher rates of injury than their male counterparts because they aren't taught to train like men. Because women have more estrogen, their ligaments and tendons are looser, so they're told to train differently to better stabilize their joints, which is completely unnecessary. Women can move weight just as heavy as men, and there are plenty of women around the world—firefighters, combat soldiers, and others—who are already proving it and breaking barriers. And they are intellectually brilliant and beautiful all at the same time. Just like my duality of being a Titan and a beauty queen, your only limits are self-imposed. To every man, boyfriend, husband, brother, and father—having a strong woman in your life is to your advantage. The pursuit of physical and athletic improvement isn't masculine, it's human. Stay hard to kill, ladies!

Chapter 5
Pillar 3: Sleep

More than Closing Your Eyes
You spend one-third of your life sleeping, so just like your waking hours, your sleep hours should be the highest quality you can have. How well you sleep determines not only how well you feel the next day but also how healthy you are. Humans are the only mammals that deliberately delay sleep. This is largely due to being overworked during the day and spending more time on devices in the evening—that fear of "missing out" and feeling the need to keep up with everyone else. But sleeping is more than just lying down and closing your eyes. You accumulate stress at a cellular level during the day and sleep is the only way your body repairs, regenerates, and syncs its schedule for the next day.

Avoiding sleep is detrimental to your health. Staying awake for more than 16 hours decreases mental and physical performance that is equivalent to having a .05% blood alcohol level (.08% is illegal in most states). Sleep requirements change with each decade of life:

Newborns: 14-17 hours

Infants: 12-15 hours

Toddlers: 11-14 hours

Preschoolers: 10-13 hours

Grade schoolers: 9-11 hours

Teens: 8-10 hours

Adults: 7-9 hours

For each hour you're awake, you need 20-30 minutes of sleep to function optimally the next day. There is a u-shaped curve that indicates how sleep correlates with health. People who regularly sleep too little—as well as too much—are at greater risk for chronic diseases such as cardiovascular disease, diabetes, and obesity. Don't let poor sleep habits shorten your life!

The Science of Sleep

How long does it take you to fall asleep at night? Sleep latency—the amount of time it takes to fall asleep—should be 10 to 20 minutes. If you can fall asleep in less than 5 minutes, it indicates you could be sleep deprived or have a sleep disorder. If it takes you longer than 30 minutes, you may have insomnia. Many things can impact sleep latency such as alcohol, pain, medication, and daytime naps. There are three levels of sleep:

Drowsy sleep: This level lasts about 10 minutes. The muscles relax, body temperature lowers, and eyes move slower as you drift off.

Light sleep: This level lasts up to 60 minutes. Your eyes stop moving, heart rate and breathing slows, and the brain rapidly fires, consolidating memories from throughout the day.

Deep sleep: This level lasts up to 40 minutes. Your blood pressure drops and heart rate slows 20-30%. The brain stops responding to stimuli, and muscle paralysis, or muscle atonia, occurs.

After passing through the first three levels, you enter the active stage of sleep, called Rapid Eye Movement (REM). During this stage, your eyes dance back and forth behind your eyelids, your breathing and heart rate speed up, your blood pressure increases, and you dream. Your first REM cycle is usually only a few minutes, but as the night progresses, each REM cycle lasts longer. These cycles are especially important for memory and learning.

Your entire sleep cycle is controlled by an area of the brain called the suprachiasmatic nucleus (SCN). It acts as the "master clock" for your body. The SCN takes signals from the presence or absence of sunlight to control systems throughout your body. It's critical to get optimal sleep to support your master clock. The reason adults need 7 hours of sleep each night is because it takes 7 hours to complete the correct number of sleep cycles. In fact, the first four hours are the most crucial. If you've ever awakened around 2 a.m., you probably felt really tired the next day as a result of interrupting your sleep cycles. As an OBGYN, delivering a baby around 2 a.m. always made it harder to function for the next couple of days.

Your circadian rhythms are the biological changes your body goes through every 24 hours. Every organ in your body is synced to your master clock, which takes its direction from the sun. Your cells, just like plants, receive and absorb light. The best night's sleep you can get starts during the day. When your body senses sunlight in the morning, it makes the hormones cortisol and insulin, which rise with the sun and help make you alert and ready to take on the day. As sunlight disappears in the evening, your body secretes a hormone called melatonin, which helps calm and relax you prior to sleep.

The sun also controls your body temperature. When your body senses sunlight, it starts to warm up. The absence of sunlight at night makes your body cool down in preparation for sleep. When you manipulate this natural temperature process, it can impact your ability to wake up or fall asleep. If you have a memory foam mattress that doesn't breathe, too many blankets, or heavy flannel pajamas, your body may not dissipate enough heat to cool down and fall asleep, leading to insomnia.

A number of factors lead to insomnia, and most of them are self-inflicted forms of ignoring the body's natural biological rhythms:

Blue light: Blue light emitted from light bulbs, computers, and smart phones stimulates the back of the eye, which signals the brain to reduce melatonin production, making you more alert, increasing your body temperature, and raising your heart rate—all things you want in the morning, not at night.

Lack of Movement: Movement and exercise help muscles secrete myokines (discussed in chapter four) and other hormones (such as melatonin) that promote sleep.

Stress: Stress increases the production of cortisol and adrenalin, which are antagonists to the sleep hormone melatonin. When your daytime cortisol and adrenalin levels are too high, it's impossible to rest and let your body repair.

Food: When you make dinner your largest meal or have a bedtime snack, your body has to work to digest that food. It pulls blood into your digestive system and heats your body, which makes it difficult to cool down and fall asleep.

Environment: Other factors such as pets in your bed, partners who snore, and loud noises outdoors can all contribute to insomnia.

Medical Conditions: Dehydration, acid reflux, obstructive

sleep apnea, and prescription medications can all be factors too.

Breathe Better, Sleep Better

When you breathe, it activates your body's nervous system—inhalation stimulates the sympathetic nervous system (known as the "fight or flight" system) and exhalation stimulates the parasympathetic nervous system (known as the "rest and digest" system). Your body uses breathing to maintain a constant state of homeostasis between these two nervous systems. Unfortunately, our society is constantly stressed, over-caffeinated, and so busy that it's in sympathetic nervous system overdrive—a constant state of "fight or flight", which isn't conducive to a good night's sleep. If you can learn to breathe properly, you'll nurture your parasympathetic nervous system, which helps reduce stress and improve sleep. Breath work is available to you every single second of the day. It is free and portable to all humans and an undervalued tool for your health.

Archeologist records show that the human mouth is shrinking. The invention of tools to cut food has resulted in less powerful teeth and smaller jaws, which impact airway development and how people breathe. Humans were designed to breathe in through the nose, not the mouth. One of the benefits infants get from breastfeeding is it helps properly form the mouth's palate and arch as well as move the airway's structures into place—babies have to breathe through their nose while breastfeeding. When children start using bottles and sippy cups too soon, it alters their oral development, can cause crowded teeth, and they turn into mouth breathers. An open mouth drops the tongue down and backward toward the throat, which can lead to snoring and sleep apnea. If you have trouble sleeping, have a professional examine your jaw, teeth, and airway for possible structural issues.

Another cause of poor sleep due to airway issues is age-related muscle loss, which was discussed in chapter four. Building muscle is important for proper breathing. When you lose muscle and gain fat, it puts pressure on your airway. Imagine your airway as a flexible garden hose. If you put rocks on top of the hose, it might not completely cut off the water, but it lessens the pressure and flow. When you put extra weight on your airway as the result of weight gain, you can't breathe as easily, which activates the sympathetic nervous system, triggers the release of cortisol and insulin, and contributes to overall metabolic disease.

Nasal breathing also increases nitric oxide, which dilates blood vessels and produces more oxygen for your tissues and cells. In turn, mouth breathing doesn't increase nitric oxide, so your body becomes stressed and fatigued. This is why oxygen saturation drops in people with sleep apnea. It doesn't matter what position you sleep in—back, side, etc.—as long as you practice breathing through your nose. I use mouth taping to help ensure nasal breathing at night. It's a safe, easy practice, and there are very good mouth tape products available on the market.

Everyone experiences times when they have trouble sleeping. But there are some easy, controllable things you can do to greatly improve your sleep hygiene and get better sleep on a regular basis. However, no amount of sleep hygiene will overcome a bad airway or medical condition such as sleep apnea.

Hard to Kill Sleep Hygiene Plan

1. *Stay cool:* Wear light, comfortable clothing, have a breathable mattress, sheets, and blankets, and keep the bedroom temperature below 70 degrees.

2. *Maintain consistency:* Create a consistent time you go to bed and wake up. Your body is on a constant clock, and it runs optimally when you perform activities such as waking, eating, and sleeping at the same times every day.

3. *Keep it quiet:* Your bedroom should only be used for sleep and sex. If you don't have control over noise outside your bedroom, invest in a fan or sound machine.

4. *Reduce blue light toxicity:* Eliminate stimulation from blue light in the evening. Turn down your

lights (you can use candlelight), change the setting on your computer, phone, or other device to reduce its blue light, wear blue-light blocking glasses, or put screen filters on your devices. There are also apps that can track how much blue light you get throughout the day so you can monitor when to reduce it.

5. *Remove electronics*: Don't have a TV in the bedroom, and place your cell phone away from your bed.

6. *No pets*: Train your pets not to sleep in bed with you at night.

7. *Smaller meals*: Don't eat within three hours of going to bed. Your largest meal should be at lunch, not at dinner.

8. *Monitor beverages*: Caffeine and alcohol can greatly affect your circadian rhythms, so be sure to limit those the closer you get to bedtime.

9. *Oral assessment*: If you think you're a mouth breather, have your dentist or another professional examine your airway, jaw, and teeth. Also consider mouth taping as a tool.

10. *Sunlight exposure*: Our eyes evolved to see a very narrow portion of the light spectrum. Upon awakening, expose your eyes to sunlight as quickly as possible. Viewing the morning sunrise for 2-3 minutes stimulates your brain to be alert.

Blue light from devices is ok in the morning but should decrease later in the day. You can also use a UV light box in parts of the world that don't get enough sunlight—anything that simulates the sun and energizes your body. Dose and duration are what matter. Alternatively, viewing the sunset's orange and red light in the evening signals your brain to relax and unwind in preparation for sleep. If you work at night, try to schedule some time during the day for sunlight exposure. And when you do sleep, even if it's primarily during daytime hours, still practice good sleep hygiene habits.

More of your energy is supplied by the sun than by food. Because your SCN gets its signals from the sun, which in turn sends appropriate signals to your brain for either energy or rest, it's critical to eliminate disruptions to your master clock. Humans are like a solar-powered light—your body uses sunlight to charge all day and then it works all night while you're asleep. Be sure that sleep is helping you become hard to kill.

Chapter 6
Pillar 4: Resilient Mindset

C ontrol Your Mind

Your brain is your greatest superpower. It can also be your biggest enemy. Everything you let enter your mind goes back out into the world—both positive and negative. Although your brain has the ability to create infinite creative thoughts and dreams, it also has a safety mechanism calibrated to ensure your survival. When it senses you may engage in a potentially dangerous activity, you have thoughts such as, "you might get hurt", "you'll lose all your money", or "people will make fun of you".

These thoughts pepper your mind, some of which you ignore and others to which you pay attention. This language either drives or prevents action in your life. You must learn to select your thoughts every single day just like you choose your clothes to wear. Your thoughts are like seeds you plant, nurture, and cultivate so you can flourish and thrive. It won't be easy, but if you want to become resilient and hard to kill, it all starts with your mind.

In the late 18th century, British physicians Alexander Sutherland and William Cullen began using placebo drugs as a way to satisfy patients who had certain expectations and demands for medical treatment. Inert substances, such as sugar pills, were given to patients who often reported feeling better after taking them. The expectation of feeling better is a key component of the placebo effect. It's not just about positive thinking but more about believing the treatment or procedure will work. Belief creates an unbreakable connection between the mind and body. There are numerous examples of this in the medical world. Patients have been given saline instead of morphine and still reported reduced pain. Surgeries have been performed in which only an incision was made and patients reported an improvement in symptoms. There have even been studies in patients with migraines who knew they received the placebo and still reported a 50% reduction in migraine pain. The placebo effect has since become the gold standard for testing new therapies because the placebo group almost always has positive results.

You can harness the power of the placebo effect and experience it in your everyday life by creating rituals. Daily habits become a driving force, and you need to establish them with all five pillars of health. It starts with sleeping well, eating well, moving well, and engaging in quality social and alone time. When you perform these rituals daily, it will foster mental, physical, and spiritual resilience. I like to call this practice non-sleep deep rest or NSDR. Doing NSDR 10-30 minutes a day, 3-7 times per week will mitigate stress in your life, improve cognition, and make you harder to kill.

Mental Resilience

Up to 95% of your behavior occurs on autopilot. Your brain receives millions of inputs and sends them down its superhighway. If you don't consciously steer those inputs in a different direction, then old, comfortable habits and behaviors will follow. It's much like driving to and from work—you don't have to think about where you're going because your brain just knows how to get there. Bad habits are almost always mindless actions that happen so quickly you don't even realize you've done them. Eating a bag of chips without realizing they're gone is a good example. Mindfulness is the ability to slow your brain and take control—essentially removing yourself from autopilot so that you are intentional with your actions and create willpower and discipline. An easy test is to drive home from work using a different route. It will make you think, engage, and adjust. Or try brushing your teeth with your non-dominant hand. Any new skill requires you to turn off autopilot. When you are more mindful, you are more intentional with your actions, which leads to better execution.

I've had countless patients describe the ways mindfulness has fundamentally changed the way they experience life. Mindfulness reduces anxiety and depression, boosts the immune system, manages pain, treats addiction, reduces blood pressure, and changes the overall function and structure of the brain. Mindfulness is the ability to be present in your life. It enables you to be aware of where you are and what you're doing in *that* moment. It also helps control your reaction to overwhelming situations. The ability to harness my mindfulness has been invaluable during times of chaos, such as when a baby I'm delivering is in trouble or a mother is bleeding out. Any physician who worked during the pandemic needed mindfulness just to endure. Mindfulness is a critical tool for survival.

When I first explored mindfulness and meditation, it was uncomfortable. I had to learn how to embrace it. Meditation forces you to explore the present moment as it is. The practice invites you into a space of sensations, emotions, and your innermost thoughts. This can be a scary place, especially for people who engage in negative self talk. If you don't know how to control those thoughts, meditation or mindfulness can feel awkward and uncomfortable. Some people fear being alone with their thoughts for this reason. But over time, this practice will strengthen your mental muscle and will help you experience more warmth and kindness toward yourself and others. It will also stimulate the brain, which changes its structure and function to help mitigate age-related cognitive decline and maintain retention, memory, and processing well into your later years.

Everyone has a large-scale brain network called the default mode network (DMN), which becomes active when you're not focused on a particular task. The DMN is usually engaged when your mind wanders, you daydream, or you're thinking about the past or future. It also plays a role in people who have attention-deficit/hyperactivity disorder (ADHD). People who regularly meditate have a less active DMN and are able to pay attention better and execute tasks with less distraction. The best part about meditation or mindfulness is that it doesn't cost anything except your time and can be done anywhere. There are numerous meditation apps you can download on your phone, but they aren't required. You can meditate or practice mindfulness with just a few simple steps.

Hard to Kill Mindfulness Exercise

1. Upon waking, sit at the edge of your bed, feet flat on the floor, and close your eyes.
2. Connect with all your sensations. What do you feel? Hear? Smell? Taste? Feel the bed underneath you. Feel the floor under your feet.

3. Place one hand on your chest and one on your stomach. Inhale through the nose for 4 seconds. Feel your stomach expand as air enters your body. Hold the breath for 4 seconds and then slowly exhale for 4 seconds, feeling your stomach lower as air leaves your body. Repeat four times.

4. When you've completed the breathing, set your intentions for the day and answer the following: "Who am I? How do I need to show up today? How can I make the biggest impact?" Positive affirmations will set your internal language, which in turn will change your next action.

5. Repeat this practice throughout the day whenever you need to be centered. You can do it at home, at the office, outdoors in the sunlight, or in a dark, quiet space.

Physical Resilience

Chapter three examined the importance of movement and physical strength, which is directly related to physical resilience. Eating adequate protein will help grow and stimulate muscles, and resistance training will stimulate autophagy, which is the body's natural process of cleaning out dead and damaged cells so it can regenerate healthy ones. When you exercise and put purposeful stress on your body, it breaks down the muscle. Helping that muscle recover will make it build back up faster so you become stronger and hard to kill.

There are many ways to support recovery and physical resilience. I am going to share with you ones that I use but this is not exhaustive. Training must be balanced with recovery. Nutrition is very important when it comes to physical recovery. Exercise and resistance training are forms of purposeful stress. The techniques discussed are also purposeful stress, but when they are performed correctly, they can make you stronger and more resilient over time. This is called "hormesis". Hormetic stress is a good thing when done properly. Just like all stress, too much will make you weak and vulnerable but just enough will make you harder to kill.

Cold Water Immersion

Cold therapy became popular in large part to Wim Hof, a Dutch extreme athlete known for his record-breaking cold exposure stunts. He has since developed the Wim Hof Method® to guide and educate about the benefits of cold therapy, which include improved cardiovascular circulation, reduced inflammation, boosted immune system, and improved metabolic health. The timing and procedure for cold water immersion therapy is important. You want to avoid cold therapy for 3-4 hours after resistance training because it can stunt muscle protein synthesis.

One of the best ways to ease into cold water immersion therapy is by taking a cold shower. Begin with your normal shower routine and water temperature. When you've finished washing, turn the water temperature as cold as you can handle and stay under it for one minute. Every day increase the amount of time you stand under the cold water until you've reached 10 minutes. When you get out of the shower, lightly towel off and then let your body rewarm via ambient air before getting dressed.

Once you are comfortable with cold showers, you can move to cold water immersion. You can do this in a bathtub or you can purchase an ice bath. Start with water that is colder than 75 degrees^F and work your way to 50-60 degrees^F or lower. Start with just a couple of minutes a few times per week. Just like with other pillars, there is an ideal length of time—if you're cold for too long, the benefits of cold therapy will start to decrease. After using cold water therapy, I've noticed faster recovery times following strenuous workouts where I'm not as sore afterward. I've experienced improvement with sleep, and I haven't been sick in nearly six years.

Your first cold plunge can be a transformative experience. I love combining it with breathing practices and mindfulness to activate the parasympathetic nervous system to combat any fight or flight thoughts and trigger nitric oxide production to stimulate oxygen in the cells. Once you immerse yourself in the ice bath, surface level blood vessels constrict and deeper blood vessels dilate to maintain body temperature. This releases norepinephrine and dopamine, which can help combat low energy, poor mood, depression, and lack of focus. There is also evidence that during cold water immersion, the body secretes cold shock proteins such as RNA-binding motif protein 3 (RBM3), which has been shown to restore and regenerate neurological synapses. This is why doctors have explored cold therapy for patients with brain and spinal injuries.

One of the major drivers for age-related chronic disease is inflammation. Studies show that 2-3 minutes of whole-body cryotherapy can reduce inflammation markers such as tumor necrosis factor alpha (TNF-a), which promotes insulin resistance and is associated with obesity-induced Type 2 diabetes, and prostaglandins, which are a group of lipids present at the site of inflammation. Cold therapy also keeps your immune system active. Lymphocytes (T cells) naturally kill virus-infected cells. It's not uncommon in other countries for parents to send their kids outside during cold weather at the onset of illness.

Another benefit of cold therapy is thermogenesis, which was mentioned in chapter three. Shivering thermogenesis occurs when you are cold and your muscles contract rapidly to keep you warm. Non-shivering thermogenesis increases brown fat metabolism to warm the body. Intermittent cold therapy leverages brown fat, which helps reduce visceral fat, combat obesity, and induces the production of antioxidants and mitochondrial biogenesis, or cell renewal. Anything that fosters healthy mitochondria in the body will make you hard to kill.

Hard to Kill Cold Water Immersion Protocol

1. You can perform cold therapy prior to exercise, but wait 3-4 hours after exercise before performing.
2. Start with a cold shower or bath with water at 75 degrees^F for 1-2 minutes. Make sure your hands and feet are submerged.
3. For each new session, lower the water temperature and increase your exposure by 1 minute until the water temperature reaches 50 degrees^F for a total exposure time of 10 minutes. If the temperature is below 50 degrees^F, then shorten the time of exposure.
4. When finished, lightly towel dry and then let ambient air rewarm you. Do not use a hot shower or sauna to warm yourself back up.
5. Perform at least 3 times per week.

Benefits:

Improved cardiovascular circulation

Reduced inflammation

Improved immune system

Reduced anxiety and depression

Improved energy

Weight loss

Improved hair and skin

Increased pain relief

Improved sleep

Reduced swelling

Improved cognitive performance

Sauna Therapy

Heat exposure is another form of purposeful stress on the body just like cold therapy and resistance training, which are all forms of hormetic stress. If you recall, hormesis is a phenomenon in which a harmful substance gives stimulating and beneficial effects to living organisms when the quantity of the harmful substance is small. In this case, small amounts of hot or cold therapy. Heat therapy also releases norepinephrine, which again helps with focus and cognitive benefits. It's interesting to note that the country with the most public saunas—Finland—also consistently ranks among the world's highest student test scores. During sauna therapy, endorphins are released, which are a natural pain killer. The therapy also regulates brain-derived neurotrophic factor

(BDNF), which helps neurons to survive and to develop new ones, especially as they are related to learning and memory. Similar to how cold therapy releases cold shock proteins, heat therapy releases heat shock proteins that act as a powerful growth hormone to increase muscle and improve cardiovascular function.

Hard to Kill Sauna Therapy Protocol

1. You can perform sauna therapy immediately after exercise or prior to cold therapy.
2. The sauna should be between 140-170 degrees^F. Start with 10 minutes of exposure as tolerated. Work up to 30-minute sessions daily.
3. When finished, wash with a gentle cleanser to remove sweat and toxins from the skin. This is very important because sweat is the primary way for the body to release toxins, chemicals, and heavy metals.
4. Drink plenty of water throughout the day to replenish electrolytes and rehydrate.

Benefits:
Decreased blood pressure
Increased muscle growth
Decreased risk of dementia

Improved cognitive performance

Improved immune system

Improved pain relief

Heavy metal detoxification

Improved skin

Reduced inflammation

Reduced anxiety and depression

Light Therapy

As discussed in chapter five, sunlight and its effect on circadian rhythms is an essential component of being hard to kill. Light is a signaling factor for all of your body's physiological processes. Depending on the wavelength and frequency, light can boost your overall health and wellness in additional ways. Natural sunlight has the following spectrums:

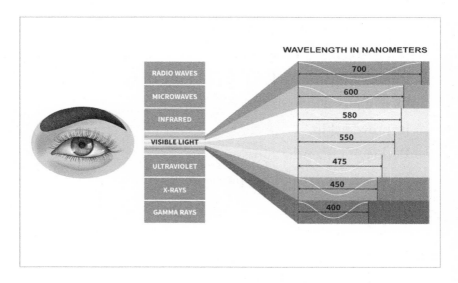

It's important to get full spectrum sunlight on a daily basis. You want the sunlight to touch your eyes just a few minutes every morning, midday, and every evening because it will help set your circadian rhythms. Sunlight is also necessary for the production of an important hormone called vitamin D. Another direct light therapy is photobiomodulation (PBM), which uses near infrared (NIR) and infrared light to stimulate cells and tissues to produce various benefits. This therapy can be administered through low level lasers, light emitting diodes, or light panels. Low level lasers were first used in the 1960s to treat wounds, improve pain, and accelerate healing and recovery. You can easily purchase red light panels and bulbs in different sizes for home use.

When skin is exposed to NIR or infrared light, it

stimulates chromophores, which promotes cellular synthesis and energy, and increases nitric oxide for improved oxygen and blood flow throughout the body. There are different types of chromophores at different depths. Infrared light wavelengths measure between 600-700 nanometers and help improve the skin's texture, tone, smooth fine wrinkles, and improve collagen. Near infrared measures between 700-1200 nanometers and penetrates deeper to help with muscle aches, joint pain, and nerve damage.

When I first started using PBM therapy, I focused on my face to help improve its overall appearance—who doesn't want a more youthful look? Then I moved down to my neck to help with thyroid production. My husband also used it as a therapy to increase testosterone production and had great success. The therapy can be performed at a doctor's office, by an esthetician, in conjunction with sauna therapy, or simply at home with a wide variety of lights from different companies. It is pain free and has no known side effects.

Hard to Kill Light Therapy Protocol (in addition to daily full-spectrum sunlight)

1. Choose an infrared light with a range of 630-660 nanometers or an NIR light with a range of 800-950 nanometers.

2. Position yourself 10-12 inches from the light (or manufacturer's recommended distance).
3. Keep your session to 10-20 minutes.
4. Perform in the morning, evening, or both. If used in the evening, do not use within 2 hours of bedtime.

Benefits
Improved pain relief
Reduced inflammation
Faster wound healing
Increased nitric oxide production
Decreased anxiety and depression
Improved nerve regeneration
Improved fat burning
Reduced cellulite
Improved stem cell production
Improved thyroid function
Improved exercise recovery
Improved testosterone production
Improved acne
Reduced fine wrinkles
Improved collagen production
Reduced hair loss
Improved sleep quality
Improved protection against macular degeneration

.   .   .

Additional Therapies

There are many other therapies available to help you achieve physical resilience. Some of these include acupuncture, cupping, dry needling, transcutaneous electrical nerve stimulation (TENS), ultrasound, and manual massage, to name a few. Exercise such as yoga and Tai Chi also provide benefits. Before starting any type of physical therapy or activity, check with your medical provider, and don't perform any therapy longer than the recommended time.

Spiritual Resilience

When something bad happens in your life, do you fall down and have a hard time getting back up, or do you bounce back quickly? Do you consider yourself to be thriving or just surviving? If you tend to struggle when faced with life's stressors, then you need to improve your spiritual resilience. Most people think of spirituality in religious contexts, and you can certainly seek spiritual strength through a higher power no matter your religious affiliations. I consider spiritual resilience the ability to maintain a positive spirit even in the face of adversity. It's the ability to draw on your own set of beliefs, principles, and values to overcome physical, intellectual, financial, and relational setbacks.

I like to think of spiritual resilience as the ripples you create in the world. When you create ripples—as I hope this book does—you connect to others through spiritual emotions such as inspiration, love, joy, hope, gratitude, compassion, and awe.

Just as the pillars discussed are connected, so is the mind, body, and spirit. You can tailor your daily rituals to heal not only your body and mind, but also your spirit, rounding out every aspect of becoming hard to kill. Prayer is one way to practice. Prayer can foster a sense of connection—with a higher power, your environment, and other people in your life.

People pray for many reasons, including guidance, gratefulness, or protection. A 2004 study on religious coping methods in the *Journal of Health Psychology* found that people who seek spiritual support and approach God as a partner in their life had better health outcomes, whereas negative methods of religious coping, such as anger or feeling punished by God, saw declines in health. And those who struggle over time may be at even greater risk for health-related problems.

Hard to Kill Spiritual Resilience Rules

1. *Be positive.* It's a fact that positive people live longer. They maintain spiritual resilience by vibrating at a higher energy level.

2. *Control the controllables.* If you can't control it, let it go, otherwise it will slowly erode your resilience.

3. *Be flexible.* Learn how to bend and not break. This will keep you more open-minded and give you the ability to adapt in all areas of your life.

4. *Respond to facts.* Be careful not to react to emotions and drama. How you respond to situations will determine if you live in fear or peace. Living in fear leads to blame and judgement, which will drive you to a negative mindset.

5. *Find your inner child.* Seek out experiences that are full of spontaneity, humor, and playfulness. They will cultivate a sense of lightheartedness and uplift your spirits as well as that of others.

6. *Find your tribe.* This may be people within your family, church, circle of friends, or other groups and organizations. Remember, you become the people with whom you spend the most time, so audit this circle often.

Chapter 7
Pillar 5: Environment

You are Your Surroundings

Your environment is probably not the first thing that comes to mind with regard to improving your health. But as you've learned throughout previous chapters, respecting nature—especially food—is incredibly important. You are the product of your surroundings—the people, places, and things you interact with on a regular basis—and all of them impact you physically, mentally, and spiritually. It's critical to have an awareness of your environment so you can periodically audit each component. It's ultimately how you build community, foster health, and become hard to kill.

Growing up, I believed that my brain and talent would be the biggest factors to contribute to my success in life. Good grades came easily, I excelled at athletics, and I was willing to sacrifice socially to attain those goals. I've always been honored to be a Division I collegiate athlete and to have earned a medical degree. But intellect and talent were only part of my success equation. I was fortunate to have an upbringing in a community of people that helped foster success. Where you live and the people you interact with are a big factor in your overall well-being.

People

Not everyone is born into the same nurturing environments. The country in the world with the longest life expectancy—Hong Kong—has an average life expectancy of more than 85 years. This is thought to be a combination of its citizens' wealth and ability to obtain excellent health care as well as access to seafood, meat, and other whole foods. Whether or not you were born in Hong Kong, born into wealth, or born into poverty, you still have the ability to choose your circle of influence over time. Ask yourself these questions about your five closest friends: Are they active? What do they eat? Do they smoke? Drink? Are they single or married? Are they positive-minded? Do they chase their dreams? Are they hard to kill? These five people have the single greatest impact on your journey and on your ability to move toward inspired action no matter where you live in the world.

There are two types of people: proactive and reactive. Reactive people waste energy—yours and theirs. They devote energy to things they can't change. They routinely gossip, complain, blame, shame, and justify their way through life. They never take responsibility for their actions. Over time, they diminish and erode others in an effort to maintain their tiny circle. They are followers, like sheep, not leaders. Being around reactive people who are disrespectful is a miserable way to spend your time. Make sure that's not how people feel about you, too.

Proactive people only expend energy on things they can control. They exude positivity and lead with a growth mindset. They make effective changes and have a large circle of influence because people are naturally attracted to them. They align themselves with people they aspire to be—those who are physically, mentally, financially, and spiritually successful.

Are you currently proactive or reactive? If you don't like the answer, the good news is you can change it. The first step in becoming hard to kill is to know which type of person you are and then align your circle of influence accordingly. A mentor of mine once gave me the following advice: if you want to own a yacht, go to the yacht club and do what the yacht owners do. Similarly, if you want to become physically fit, spend time with a physically fit person and follow their routine. Being proactive simply comes down to the execution of daily habits.

When I speak with patients whose goal is to eat healthier, work out, quit smoking, or eliminate the need for medications,

I always ask them about the relationships in their life. If they have a spouse or close friend who doesn't align with their goal, I can almost always bet the bank in Vegas they won't be able to achieve or sustain it. No success is ever accomplished alone. As you set out on your hard to kill journey, you need to routinely audit your circle of influence. The people in your circle should be able to name your physical, intellectual, and financial goals, and you should be able to name theirs. These are the relationships you need to build. As you assess your circle, eliminate drama, refuse negativity, reject toxicity, and remove anyone with habits you don't want for yourself. Creating distance from someone may require a new school, job, or partner. It can be difficult to make that change, but life is short. Don't forget that time is your most valuable asset. Positive thinking can extend your life by 11-15% regardless of age, gender, income, or location. Maintaining a positive outlook while surrounded by optimistic people will help you become hard to kill.

Places

Not only is it important to surround yourself with the right people, but equally important is the space you occupy with them. There are areas of the world that have extreme longevity—little pockets where people seem to be harder to kill. These areas are called Blue Zones® because researchers drew blue circles around the locations on a map. Scientists have studied the areas in an attempt to find the lifestyle habits the people in each zone have in common. Dan Buettner, Blue Zones® founder, discovered five places in the world where people live the longest and are the healthiest: Okinawa, Japan; Sardinia, Italy; Nicoya, Costa Rica; Ikaria, Greece, and Loma Linda, California. It appears longevity is the result of a constellation of small things that help these humans thrive for a long time. They eat whole foods, do a lot of walking, and most importantly engage in deep human connection within their communities. Sound like a familiar plan?

Places with the Longest Life Expectancy according to World Population Review (listed in years):

1. *Hong Kong:* 84.9
2. *Japan:* 84.67
3. *Macau:* 84.396
4. *Switzerland:* 83.836
5. *Singapore:* 83.662
6. *Spain:* 83.612
7. *Italy:* 83.568
8. *Australia:* 83.496
9. *Iceland:* 83.07

Places with the Lowest Life Expectancy, according to World Population Review (listed in years):

1. *Central African Republic:* 53.345 *years*

2. *Chad: 54.458*

3. *Lesotho: 54.366*

4. *Nigeria: 54.808*

5. *Sierra Leone: 54.81*

6. *Somalia: 57.5*

7. *Ivory Coast: 57.844*

8. *South Sudan: 57.948*

9. *Guinea Bissau: 58.444*

The 2022 life expectancy in the United States is currently at 78.999 years—6 fewer years than Hong Kong. The two biggest factors for life expectancy are genetics and lifestyle, so where you live can affect your health. Your genes are like a light switch and your environment is what turns them on or off. You do have the ability to influence your potential through epigenetics. The way you interact with your environment modifies your gene expression without altering the genetic code itself. Smoke, air pollution, electromagnetic fields, soil, and water quality all play a part. The things you are exposed to can alter your microbiome and impact your health. The WHO estimates that 12 million people die every year due to environmental risk factors that drive heart disease, respiratory disease, and some cancers. I can't solve the world's pollution problems, but it's important to acknowledge the impact it has on your health and that where you live in the world matters.

Water is essential for life. The WHO estimated that in 2020 only 74% of the world population had access to a safely managed water source. That means one in four people don't have access to safe drinking water. The WHO also estimated that 2 billion people globally use drinking water contaminated with feces and 829,000 deaths occur annually from contaminated drinking water. Chemicals such as lead, arsenic, nitrates, and nitrites are often found in water supplies. According to the Environmental Protection Agency (EPA) it is estimated there are between 6 and 10 million lead service water lines in the U.S. Lead exposure can cause anemia, weakness, infertility, kidney and brain damage. There's a long list of places in the U.S. where chemicals have been found in water supplies—arsenic in central California, radium in Texas, and copper in Michigan, to name a few.

The bigger emerging problems now are contaminants in the water such as pharmaceuticals, pesticides, per-and polyfluoroalkyl substances (PFAS) and perfluorooctanoic acid (PFOA). These chemicals are used to make fluoropolymer coatings that resist heat, stains, oil, and grease and are used in products such as clothing, furniture, adhesives, food packaging, and heat-resistant non-stick cooking surfaces. They are problematic because they don't break down in the environment, easily contaminate drinking water sources, and build up in fish and wildlife. Exposure to water, food, and products contaminated with PFAS can lead to health problems such as thyroid disease, liver damage, decreased fertility, and cancer.

During my pediatrics rotation as a medical student, I was pregnant with my first daughter. While performing rounds with other physicians, a pediatric cardiothoracic surgeon saw me drinking water out of a store-bought plastic bottle. He said he couldn't watch me take another drink and gently removed it from my hand and threw it in the trash can. He went on to explain that he'd spent the past several years operating on newborns with congenital heart conditions, many of whom came from a particular part of the state. He was convinced it was due to chemical runoff in the water supply of these farming communities. Water in plastic bottles also leaches chemicals even if the water originally bottled was pure. That moment had a lasting impact on me, and to this day, I only drink filtered water and never out of a plastic bottle. You should pay attention to your water source and do everything you can to make it safer to drink to protect you and your family.

Things

Muscle is the largest organ with regard to weight, but skin wins with regard to surface area, which makes it the best organ to absorb everything it touches. This includes clothing, soap, lotion, sunscreen, cosmetics, medications, and more. The gastrointestinal tract also has a large surface area and capacity for absorption. One of the reasons I'm so passionate about the things we put in and on our bodies is because as an OBGYN, I take care of women and their babies who are especially vulnerable.

In a study commissioned by the Environmental Working . Group (EWG), umbilical cord blood was studied in minority babies. Of the more than 400 chemicals tested, 287 were detected in umbilical cord blood of all the babies tested. Of the 287 chemicals, 180 cause cancer in humans or animals, 217 are toxic to the brain and nervous system, and 208 cause birth defects or abnormal development in animal tests. Among the chemicals, eight were perfluorinated compounds (PFC), which are active ingredients or byproducts of Teflon™, fabric and carpet protectors, and food wrap coatings. Of the more than 40,000 chemicals used in the U.S., fewer than 1% have been tested for human safety, according to the EPA. Bisphenol A (BPA), is one of the biggest chemical offenders. It's found in receipt paper, food and beverage can liners, food packaging, toys, and water bottles. Retail receipts and plane tickets printed at the airport kiosk are dangerous to your health. If you use alcohol-based hand sanitizer before touching them, your BPA absorption is ten-fold. Manufacturers have now removed BPA only to replace them with similar chemicals, so don't be fooled. Cosmetics are another group known for hazardous chemicals. The word "fragrance" or "flavoring" could mean dozens of harmful substances. Rather than panic about what may be unavoidable exposures in your daily life, focus on a strategy to reduce chemicals when possible.

Hard to Kill Healthy Environment Plan

1. *Make your own cleaning products.* Things like vinegar, water, and baking soda are safe, effective cleaners.

2. *Avoid fragrance.* This includes perfumes and colognes as well as plug-in air fresheners, scented candles, scented lotions, soaps, detergents, or personal care products. Also avoid scented dryer sheets. Instead, use a natural wool ball with essential oils.

3. *Avoid plastics.* Switch to drinking and eating only from glass or stainless steel. Never heat food in a plastic container or drink hot beverages out of plastic or Styrofoam cups. Switch all food storage to glass containers and only use cookware that is glass, ceramic, cast iron, or stainless steel. Some nonstick coatings are derived from harmful substances.

4. *Avoid printed receipts and airline tickets.* Have them emailed instead.

5. *Avoid canned foods.* Many cans are lined with BPA and other chemicals, so be careful when

choosing products. Select fresh or frozen fruits and vegetables instead. Store food in glass jars when necessary.

6. *Cleaner cosmetics*. Look for makeup, cleansers, lotions, and soaps with fewer chemicals. Use natural sunscreens that provide a physical barrier (such zinc oxide sunscreens) rather than a chemical barrier.

7. *Reduce disinfectant products*. Don't buy products or clothing with the word "antibacterial" because they are likely to contain extra chemicals like triclosan—a known carcinogen.

8. *Remove shoes at the door*. Your shoes bring chemicals, oils, and contaminants into your living space. Place rugs by doors and provide shoe storage. Clean your floors regularly. Choose solid surface floors instead of carpet when possible.

9. *Add live plants to your living space*. Plants are a great way to naturally purify air. They can remove formaldehyde, xylene, benzine, and toluene chemicals that enter spaces through cleaners and synthetic building materials. Some of my favorite plants are spider plants and mother in laws tongue.

10. *Find clean water*. Use the Environmental Work Group water filter guide online and never drink out of plastic bottles.

11. *Avoid pesticides and fertilizers.* If working outdoors, remove shoes when entering your home and shower immediately so you don't track these chemicals indoors.

12. *Check your vacuum.* Make sure it contains a HEPA filter or consider a home air purification system.

13. *Wash fruits and vegetables.* You can make your own fruit and vegetable wash using 1 cup vinegar, 4 cups filtered water, and a splash of lemon juice.

14. *Pay attention to food labels.* Artificial food dyes, preservatives, and other chemicals are prevalent in all processed foods. Master Pillar 1 by eating whole foods and this won't be an issue.

15. *Pay attention to clothing labels.* Avoid clothing, bed sheets, and undergarments that contain polyester, rayon, acrylic, and nylon. The chemicals and plastics in these fibers have been shown to cause infertility, emit pollution, cause skin issues, and allergies. Choose organic cotton when possible.

16. *Avoid toxic people.* Perform routine audits of your circle to ensure you surround yourself with people who will help set you up for success.

Chapter 8
Hard to Kill 30-Day Challenge

The 5 Pillars in Action

Now that you're familiar with all five pillars, it's time to put them together into one plan, and that can only happen through action. You need to start now without hesitation. The best way to do that is through a 30-day challenge, which enables you to address all five pillars at once. Some pillars will be easier than others, but don't overthink it or obsess over any one pillar. It will be an evolution of your health journey that may look different year to year. Since 2015, my family and I have been slowly adopting everything discussed in this book. Through time and perseverance, you will become stronger. Everyone has a different DNA, and what works for me may not work for you. But you will figure out how to be an expert about your own body. You will form new habits, become resilient, and become an entirely different human being. If it seems too overwhelming to address all five pillars at once, you can focus on just one. Pillar 1 is a great place to start because nutrition is something that you must consider every day, usually multiple times per day. But don't sacrifice the other four pillars for a single super strong pillar. Eventually you'll have to make them all equally strong. Don't strive for perfection; consistency is what gets results. Remember, your life won't change until you change your mind.

Hard to Kill 30-day Challenge: NON-NEGOTIABLE

- 7 hours of sleep daily
- 5 minutes of morning sunlight exposure directly to your eyes
- 10 breaths upon awakening: 4-second inhalation through your nose, 4 seconds holding your breath, 4-second exhalation through your mouth
- Read aloud the Hard to Kill manifesto (below) to yourself in the mirror daily
- Eat a whole food diet: 30 grams of protein 3 times day, and no more than 30 grams of carbohydrates daily; prioritize protein, then fill with fat and count your carbs
- 45-minute workout daily, and prioritize resistance training

- 15 -minute walk outdoors daily, rain or shine
- Drink only water, nothing else
- Always take the stairs
- 5 minutes of evening sunlight exposure directly to your eyes
- Repeat breathing exercise before bedtime
- Follow the Hard to Kill Healthy Environment Plan

Follow this plan for 30 days in a row. If you skip any steps or fall off the plan, you must start over. Mistakes made more than once are choices. Once you've successfully completed the 30-day challenge, you can start to incorporate other features discussed from the five pillars, but don't forget to continue to follow the 30-day challenge as outlined. Keep it simple, do not overthink it. Excellence does not happen by accident. It comes from effort, knowledge, and precise execution of the plan. You must see obstacles as opportunities. You can also use the online Hard to Kill Academy as a source for additional education and ideas.

Hard to Kill Community

You are not in this alone. You have a group—a tribe, a squad, a collection of people united in the pursuit of becoming hard to kill. We will support each other in this endeavor. I encourage you to recruit others to participate with you in the Hard to Kill 30-day Challenge. You'll quickly discover who is merely interested in what you're doing and who is truly committed to this new way of living. As you master your new lifestyle, not everyone in your circle will be ready to join you. This doesn't mean you have to change who you are or what you're doing, but you may need to separate yourself or let go of those people not ready or willing to accompany you on your journey. I experienced this when I first started incorporating changes in 2015. Even to this day, there are people who want me to fail. You will find that others' insecurities will get projected on you as you outgrow them. Confidence is created through action. Don't ever apologize for your confidence, even if it offends insecure people. Make a declaration that you deserve a circle of friends who are healthy, prosperous people. Greatness is the ability to inspire those around you. Let your results speak for themselves. You are not responsible for saving anyone but yourself.

As a physician, I know from experience you can't convince people to improve. You can only lead by example, which is why I wrote this book. I want to walk this walk with you, not just as a leader in the medical community, but as a fellow human trying to strive to be my best. Being hard to kill is not what you do; it is who you are. There are more than 8 billion people in the world and many are ready to meet you at your level of commitment. I encourage you to join our online community at doctorfitandfabulous.com and use the social media tags #hardtokill #hardtokill30 and #iamhardtokill when you share your progress on social media. I've also created the following Hard to Kill manifesto for you to recite and follow as you start your journey:

Hard to Kill Manifesto:
    I am on this earth for a purpose.
    Every day that I wake up is a great day.
    I will embrace discomfort.
    Where I spend my time and energy defines my existence.
    I will respect my body.
    I have no excuses.
    I create my own happiness.
    I want my life and no one else's.
    I value my health.
    I will routinely audit my circle.
    I am responsible for my actions, not outcomes.
    My life will inspire others.
    I will honor my word.
    I will be resilient.
    I am hard to kill.

Conclusion

The one guarantee we have in life is death, so I want you to write your own story for how you'd like to spend whatever time you have left on this earth. You have the pen—it's up to you. How can your story impact others? You need to respect yourself and stop wasting time on things you're not committed to doing. Show up for yourself every day like it's the most important event on your schedule. It will be incredible to watch how your world changes once you take responsibility for everything in your life. Remember, every thought that enters your mind will manifest itself in your life. I hope you can use the 5 pillars of health to create an unshakable foundation. Complexity is the enemy of execution, so keep your plan simple. You'll face many choices —both internal and external—as you tackle your new life, but I know you can do it. I know you will become hard to kill.

Final Thoughts and the Future of Medicine

I approached this book simply as a fellow human being. I purposely didn't cite 1,000s of articles and try to sound like the authority on information. I only know what is true today based on the information I have at my disposal and my personal experience. I can assure you I have an open mind. I am willing to look, listen, and logically consider all information. I am more interested in finding the truth than I am in being right. I'm not sure where medicine is headed. I know in my heart that many people can be healed with this hard to kill plan. If we get back to the basics, our doctors and scientists can continue to advance technology in more important areas and spend less time on a self-perpetuating chronic disease Ferris wheel. Unfortunately, there is a lot of money to be made in "sick care". In the U.S. we have a high-cost system with poor outcomes. Let this be a warning: our system is on the road to implosion and you are going to need to save yourself.

By age 65, almost every American has two diseases. These patients bounce from specialist to specialist and no one is addressing why they developed the problems in the first place. It's all about volume when it comes to fee for service. This means we have to see more and more patients, spending less and less time addressing their problems. Doctors are suffering from moral injury. Most of us entered medicine because we believed it was an honorable art. In reality it is a "turn and burn" approach with less decision-making capacity.

Doctors and other health care providers are burnt out, over worked, and expected to "fix" a patient in 10 minutes. Doctors do not get paid for writing prescriptions. We want to help patients. We just don't have the correct tools.

There is also a large disconnect between doctors and scientists. On an academic level, many ideas that are studied don't always translate into clinical practice. Mice studies don't always translate to humans. Study design is sometimes poor. Sometimes research is funded by people with bias and power. Even quality studies can take an average of 17 years to translate into clinical practice. I don't have time to wait and neither do you. The internet's ability—especially social media —to rapidly disseminate information has helped shorten this time frame, as we saw during the COVID-19 pandemic. This may be for better or for worse. Who should decide what is good information or misinformation?

Patients are now more knowledgeable than ever. It's not uncommon for patients to bring me peer reviewed studies. Unfortunately, evidence-based medicine can be tainted by special interest groups, money, and corruption. Patients and doctors don't know who to trust sometimes. The nutrition policy propaganda discussed in chapter two still takes place today. I have high hopes for the dietary guidelines being drafted for 2025, but to be honest, I will not hold my breath.

Scientific productivity is measured by the number of publications and citations in research rather than its quality. Researchers should be rewarded based on their ability to replicate results that translate into helping people achieve better outcomes. Research is expensive, and society has allowed the pharmaceutical industry to fund most clinical trials and publish them under the names of senior academic officials. I fear we will lose the integrity of science if this continues. We have an industry that owns data and knowledge and can hide negative trial outcomes, fail to report adverse events, and withhold data from the rest of the academic community. As a result, patients will—and have —died.

What can you do to help? You can control your thoughts, actions, and beliefs. If you master the 5 Pillars of Health, you will need less medicine. One of my goals is to live to be 100 years old. There are incredible scientists studying how to increase longevity, and regenerative medicine is the future. I have started to mold my medical practice in this direction and opened a first-of-its-kind facility in 2021 called Upgrade Performance Institute. We use cutting-edge technology such as artificial intelligence resistance equipment, DEXA body scanners, IV nutritional therapy, NAD+ coenzymes, peptides, stem cells, exosomes, and more.

However, even if you master the 5 Pillars of Health, you can't avoid death. Researchers have many theories as to why people can't live forever and have discovered that humans have stem cell exhaustion, epigenetic changes, and telomere attrition. The study of longevity is exploding, and I'm actively learning, reading, listening, and practicing in that space.

There are case reports of genetic therapy, which uses CRISPR technology to edit a person's genes—maybe you and I can both live to be 100 years old.

There are always trade-offs, and I am a believer that you can't completely alter nature. Gene editing may turn out to be a total disaster. Humans are biological creatures that started as one singular cell. In the human egg, or oocyte, there are 600,000 mitochondria—more than any other cell in your body—that serve as sensors to the outside world, communicating with your genetic code. Your DNA code is passed down time after time, but only after it receives information from your nutrition, movement, sleep, stress, sunlight, and environment during your lifetime. These sensing pathways are a requisite for life.

The 5 Pillars of Health make you hard to kill because they impact your DNA. The choices you make right now have epigenetic influences that are passed to eggs and sperm, which will impact your family tree forever. Will you be a solid or weak branch? As an OBGYN, I am fascinated every time I deliver a baby and see a new genetic symphony born right before my eyes. I never know how much time they will have on earth or what they may achieve, but the possibilities are endless. Maybe one day they will read this book and become one more person who is hard to kill.

Acknowledgments

To my husband Ben, your love and support on this crazy path is never unnoticed. I'm grateful for what we have built together, forever and always.

To my girls Breklyn, Sienna, and Kimber. You are all one of a kind, unique, and worthy of this amazing life. Embrace every ounce of your strength and realize your time, energy, and health are your most valuable assets. I broke the mold for you to build your own authentic lives, and I cannot wait to watch them unfold.

To Mom and Dad, thank you for giving me life and all the lessons it teaches. Your baby girl will make you proud.

To Jay for your constant encouragement in writing this book.

To Matt and Bob for always capturing my story in the best light.

To Dan, our story would not be possible without you, we are forever grateful.

To Judy and Rick, thank you for your daughter, your love, and support.

To Kathy, for making this gynecologist become an author.

Selected References

Pillar 1: Nutrition

Association, A.D. (2019). *Key Takeaways from ADA's Nutrition Consensus Report.* American Diabetes, Association.

Joseph JJ, Deedwania P, Acharya T, Aguilar D, Bhatt DL, Chyun DA, Di Palo KE, Golden SH, Sperling LS; on behalf of the American Heart Association Diabetes Committee of the Council on Lifestyle and Cardiometabolic Health; Council on Arteriosclerosis, Thrombosis and Vascular Biology; Council on Clinical Cardiology; and Council on Hypertension. Comprehensive management of cardiovascular risk factors for adults with type 2 diabetes: a scientific statement from the American Heart Association.

Circulation.   2022;145:e722–e759.   doi: 10.1161/CIR.0000000000001040

Agriculture., U. D. (2015). *2015–2020 Dietary Guidelines for Americans.* Retrieved from http://health.gov/ dietaryguidelines/2015/guidelines/

Astrup A, M. F. (2020). A Reassessment and Proposal for Food-based Recommendations. *Journal of American College of Cardiology.*

Cristin E. Kearns, D. M. (2016). Sugar Industry and Coronary Heart Disease Research. *JAMA Internal Medicine.*

Select Committee on Nutrition and Human Needs, U. S. (1977). *Dietary Goals for the United States.* Washington, D.C.

Staff, H. H. (2022, January 19). *How Much Protein do you Need Every Day?* Retrieved from Harvard Health: https:// www.health.harvard.edu/blog/how-much-protein-do-you- need-every-day-201506188096

Statistics, N. C. (2018). *National Health and Nutrition Examination Survey.* Centers for Disease Control and Prevention.

Sylvan LeeWeinberg MD, M. (2004). The diet–heart hypothesis: a critique. *Journal of the American College of Cardiology*, 731-733.

World Health Organization. (2021, June 9). Retrieved from https://www.who.int/news-room/fact-sheets/detail/obesity-and-overweight

Horne BD, May HT, Muhlestein JB, *et al* Association of periodic fasting with lower severity of COVID-19 outcomes in the SARS-CoV-2 prevaccine era: an observational cohort from the INSPIRE registry *BMJ Nutrition, Prevention & Health* 2022;

Pillar 2: Movement

Jones C.J., Rikli R.E., Beam W.C.: A 30-s Chair-Stand Test to Measure Lower Body Strength in Community-Residing Older Adults. *Journal of Aging & Physical Activity,* Jan 2000;

(2019, May 1). Retrieved from Harvard Health: https://www.health.harvard.edu/staying-healthy/more-push-ups-may-mean-less-risk-of-heart-problems

Staff, H. H. (2016, February 19). *Harvard Health.* Retrieved from https://www.health.harvard.edu/staying-healthy/preserve-your-muscle-mass

Pillar 3: Sleep

(2021, September 23). Retrieved from sleep.com: https://www.sleep.com/sleep-health/how-many-hours-of-sleep

(2021, February 1). Retrieved from Healthline.com: https://healthline.com/health/nose-breathing

Pillar 4: Resilient Mindset

R., J. (2013 Apr;21(2):94-7.). The early history of the placebo. *Complement Ther Med.*

Hahn, K. I. (2004). Religious Coping Methodsd as Predictors of Psychological, Physical and Spiritual Outcomes among Medically Ill Elderly Patients: a Two-year Longitudinal Study. *Journal of Health Psychology*, 713-730.

Pillar 5: Environment

(n.d.). Retrieved from Wim Hof Method: https://www.wimhofmethod.com/

(n.d.). Retrieved from United States Environmental Protection Agency: https://www.epa.gov/ground-water-and-drinking-water/lead-service-line-replacement

(2009, November 23). Retrieved from Environmental Working Group: https://www.ewg.org/research/pollution-minority-newborns

(2016, March 15). Retrieved from World Health Organization: https://www.who.int/news/item/15-03-2016-an-estimated-12-6-million-deaths-each-year-are-attributable-to-unhealthy-environments

(2022, March 21). Retrieved from World Health Organization: https://www.who.int/news-room/fact-sheets/detail/drinking-water

Blue Zones. (n.d.). Retrieved from https://www.bluezones.com/

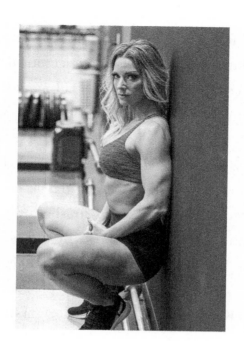

About the Author

Dr. Jaime Seeman is a board-certified Obstetrician and Gynecologist. Born and raised in Nebraska, she played collegiate softball for the University of Nebraska Cornhuskers. She has a Bachelor of Science degree in Nutrition, Exercise and Health Sciences. Dr. Seeman graduated medical school and completed her OBGYN residency at the University of Nebraska Medical Center. She is highly skilled in obstetrics, gynecology, robotic surgery, nutrition, and primary care. Dr. Seeman is fellowship trained in Integrative Medicine at the University of Arizona College of Medicine. She is a board-certified ketogenic nutrition specialist through the American Nutrition Association. She has a passion for fitness, preventative medicine, and low carb therapy not only in her medical practice but in her own life. She is the co-medical director of Upgrade Performance Institute, a first of its kind facility where muscle meets medicine. She speaks internationally and is a trusted expert in her field. She is married to her husband, Ben, a former police sergeant and has three young daughters. Dr. Seeman was also Mrs. Nebraska 2020, finished top 15 at Mrs. America 2021, and appeared on NBC's *The Titan Games* with Dwayne "The Rock" Johnson, debuting in 2020.

Visit Hard to Kill Academy: www.doctorfitandfabulous.com.

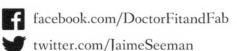

facebook.com/DoctorFitandFab

twitter.com/JaimeSeeman

instagram.com/doctorfitandfabulous

youtube.com/DoctorFitandFabulous

Made in the USA
Las Vegas, NV
11 September 2022